Healthcare Hawaii Style

Visit www.booksurge.com to order additional copies.

Healthcare Hawaii Style

Model For The Nation?

How The Aloha State Leads The Way Toward
Universal Health Care

Frank L. Tabrah, MD

2007

Healthcare Hawaii Style

TABLE OF CONTENTS

PREFACE

Why do otherwise harmless people write books? Humor suggests boredom, vanity, or money, but there is more—the wish to share an understanding that may come in a flash, or take a lifetime to emerge.

This is the story of 200 years of medical history in Hawaii, its roots lying largely in our plantation culture, shaped by epidemics, economic crises, mass migrations, powerful labor union forces, and at least since WWII, the rare bounty of intercultural amity.

Throughout the years, Hawaiian values of charity and forbearance, together with the rational pragmatic nature of our Asian population, have created a state health system with generous insurance plans and public health services that might well serve as a model for a national universal health service.

From the early 1800s, Hawaiian kings, physicians, nurses, and government have provided for competent care in our isolated island world.

With the social and economic successes of the later plantation years, health professionals, in moving from field labor beginnings to the halls of power, have retained the basic human values of the plantation communities. These communities, throughout the islands, were in later years models of thrift, vision, productivity, and major corporate support.

"Local" cooperation that melds Hawaiian compassion with the practical values of our interdependent population has spawned our unusually successful state healthcare system, shaping its rural hospital programs, strong public health commitments, and nearly universal insurance coverage.

Although today, while Hawaii shares with the nation falling Federal support for its medical services, few patients here go untreated, just as in the last fifty years of plantation life when the state, county, and employers generously paid for community health needs.

Nostalgia can be harnessed to preserve the best from the past. Our story relives the unique history in Hawaii of the truly universal healthcare available from dedicated physicians and their supporters in industry and public health. A national universal, single-pay system could well follow its lead.

This complex tale of the growth of essentially full health coverage in Hawaii stems from my own seventeen years experience as a plantation physician, later time in our clinics, laboratories, and university halls, and from many sources to which I have tried to give full credit, some of it paraphrased, and some quoted directly.

Because of my work with the John A. Burns School of Medicine Department of Pharmacology through our mutual interest in "Hawaiian Medicine", and particularly, strong public interest in it, I have included a summary of our entire natural products search in Appendix I, with some conclusions about Alternative Medicine uses in Hawaii which may serve to invite further detailed study of plant or sea materials.

I thank Chris Lothian of Hilo, Hawaii, who envisioned this book over twenty years ago, Dr. Emily Friedman (Assistant Professor of Bioethics, Boston University School of Public Health), Mr. Clifford Cisco (Senior Vice President of Hawaii Medical Service Association), Eleanor C. Nordyke, and Dr. Donald Berwick of the Harvard School of Public Health.

Stephanie Whalen, President of the Hawaii Agricultural Research Center, and Ann Marsteller, Librarian, provided gracious assistance in the use of their extensive library, for which I am most grateful.

I also wish to thank the staff members of the University of Hawaii Hamilton Library, the Department of Land and Natural Resources, State of Hawaii, Maile Drake at the Bishop Museum and Mary Anne Maigret at the State of Hawaii Department of Land and Natural Resources, for their assistance, and Ms. Evelyn Clark for information about Dr. James Wight's Kohala estate.

Mr. Jerry Walker and Mr. Kelly Roberson of Hawaii Health Systems Corporation kindly provided needed facts about Hawaii's State hospitals.

Dr. Kenneth Robbins of Straub Clinic and Hospital provided valuable office space and computer support during the preparation of this book; Debbie Bonser, of Straub Clinic and Hospital repeatedly squelched the devils in my computer, and my wife, Ernestine Tabrah, was awesome as a critic and expert in assembling information and photographs. Any errors are mine, for which I apologize.

May this book entertain you and bring to life Hawaii's unique medical past. Proponents of National Health plans and single-party payment systems will find much in the universal coverage of the plantation years and the success of mandatory health coverage since 1974 to ponder in solving our health care crisis.

FLT

Photo Credits:

I thank the Hawaiian Historical Society of Honolulu, Hawaii, for use of the photographs on pages 16, 17, 20, 21, 22 (upper) and 23, (upper). I also thank the Lyman House Memorial Museum in Hilo, Hawaii, for use of the photographs on pages 80 and 81 from their 1985 publication, The Private Japanese Hospital.

The Hawaiian Agricultural Research Center graciously provided the photographs on pages 35, 49-55, 57, 59, 71, and 72.

I thank Queen's Medical Center of Honolulu, Hawaii for the photos on pages 22 and 23, (lower).

CHAPTER I

Kohala, Hawaii

Picture the scene—1956, a highly specialized doctor, a stranger fresh from a mainland pediatric practice, a "haole" or Caucasian, on a lush tropical evening, settling into a Victorian-built "manager's house"—dizzy with the day's whirl of new people, wondrous pidgin words, exotic flowers, new foods—the mystery of it all in new scents, burning cane smelling like hot cookies, a whiff of neighbor Kimo Bowman's pigs on the soft Kona wind, all in the whirl of anticipation of a brand new Hawaii island lifestyle. My family and I had finally arrived at the village where another physician was badly needed on a booming 13,000-acre sugar plantation at the north tip of Hawaii Island in the Hawaiian Archipelago.

I had just come home from the tiny frame plantation clinic that was to be my office for seventeen magic years—household furniture was to arrive tomorrow from Hilo on a molasses truck bed, if the sea-swept barge arrived on schedule. It was a typical clinic day, a mélange of some fifty patients, welcoming leis and endless good wishes, when up our driveway from the adjacent park came a speeding WWII jeep carrying a very anxious man with his pig-hunting dog lying in the back, missing about a fourth of one side of his rugged doggy chest, showing a fair bit of bleeding lung, the worse for a tangle with a wild boar. What to do?

Little then did I know of the hundred-plus years of plantation-physician history that began in the early 1800s before the first missionaries arrived, when the first truly commercial sugar-producing effort began on Lanai in 1802 by a Chinese gentleman named Wong Tzu Chun who grew and ground one crop and returned to China.

Dozens of other bold seekers of fortune tried in ensuing years to establish small and large plantations, mostly led by foreigners, primarily missionaries, and Hawaiian leaders. Profitable yields at Pearl Harbor and Manoa Valley on Oahu, Wailuku on Maui, and Koloa on the island of Kauai, led to the flurry of planting and machinery development that became our nearly two hundred year bonanza. Mills were built, ox, horse, human, and water powered, dismantled and moved again and again. Production was more determined by luck and weather than plan. Disease (plant and human), land availability, and market price of sugar controlled success or failure. Most of all, the health of workers would determine the future.

But back to our damaged doggy. No veterinarian was within hundreds of miles. "Surgery" was the word, but dare we go to the plantation hospital? I had only met the supervisor that morning, a frowning but delightful old-school nurse who doubled as anesthetist as needed, dribbling ether out of a can onto the patient's gauze mask. Would a dog fit into her world of clinical propriety? We took no chances. Doggy, his owner and I, entering the old frame building through back passages, fired up the OR with its 1900s shiny multi-mirrored lamp with bull's eye lenses, found instruments (unsterilized), sutures and went full ahead (damn the torpedoes) to fix our patient. Dog owner, as assistant, did well, dog likewise. With a large dose of Penicillin, and wrapped up like a mummy in gauze, my patient went home. "Discharge planning" lay far in the future.

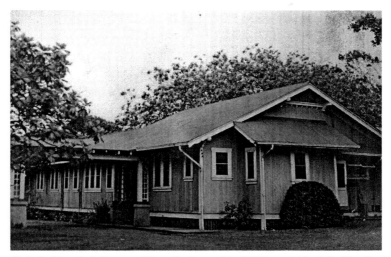

Kohala Hospital, Kapaau, Hawaii. Opened in 1917 as a 14 bed facility "in charge of" an Australian nurse. Hospitalization rate was $ 1.50 a day. The building was replaced in 1962.

Next day, I drove out to visit my patient in his kennel. We still made house calls in those days. Armed with a large empty syringe and a long needle, I expected to have to drain fluid from the dog's chest, or least some air. When I arrived, doggy was out playing in the yard with his peers—no chest fluid, no air, and no infection, nothing, and was back hunting pigs in three weeks.

With this bit of clinical good luck, and the neighbor's local pidgin comment, "haole doc, OK though," I began what was to become years of idyllic plantation practice amid a microcosm of energetic productivity, overlaid with a surprising level of racial and cultural harmony.

On Hawaii's plantations, a closer look at the relationships of our richly diversified population with the physicians, nurses, and health care assistants that served them in a universal pre-paid care system reveals an intriguing medical history, one that in good times and bad, was threaded through with the light of aloha and *ohana*, the Hawaiian ideals of family and community cooperation, principles that made life better for thousands of workers.

Nearly all of the sugar and pineapple plantations have closed, but vivid memories of the astounding productivity of workers at every level, and of the work ethic they practiced remain. Studies of the business side of the plantations have uncovered a world of imagination, risk, failure, altruism, greed, profit and disaster among owners and managers, but from our vantage point, we see that the plantation communities thrived by a paternalism that led to decades of some of the most generous and effective public health advances anywhere in the world.

Excellent medical care was provided, without billings, fees, or dunning for payments. How could all of this have worked so well, for so many years, and is there any lesson in it for today's national health care coverage gap of forty five million people?

CHAPTER 2

Early Beginnings

Who were the earliest plantation workers and who cared for them? Foreigners as planters, and native Hawaiian laborers were the first sugar producers. Although Hawaiian practitioners for many centuries had provided the bulk of medical care for their people, some of the missionary companies that arrived between 1820 and 1849 had physicians among them who treated everyone.

The first true "plantation physician" was Dr. Thomas Lafon, a physician and preacher, born in Virginia, who came around the Horn to Honolulu in 1837. The missionaries assigned him to Kauai as "resident physician," with reasonable expectations that he could work as physician for the new Ladd and Company plantation at Koloa, Kauai.

William Ladd, William Hooper, and Peter Brinsdale, were three young entrepreneurs from Boston, who, after first forming a mercantile trade company in Honolulu in 1835, settled in Koloa and set about establishing a sugar plantation. They took a fifty-year lease on 980 acres, which by 1836 they had developed into 250 acres of cane, 20 laborers' houses, shops, a dam, mill and boiling house. Their dual interests were to provide hard work for the Hawaiian people, and to make money.

Unfortunately, not all was peace and quiet at Ladd and Company. Lafon, a strong abolitionist, came to Hawaii already angered by his mission's acceptance of support from southern slave owners. Rejecting missionaries in general, he left Kauai in 1841 and Hawaii permanently in 1842. His employers, Ladd and Hooper, and their missionary friends had other problems too, as reported by historians William. H. Dorance and Francis. S. Morgan, in their 2000 Book, *Sugar Islands*, a landmark of Hawaiian history.

Of Hooper and Ladd, they write:

> *"Hooper's initial efforts to hire Hawaiian workers were met with fierce resistance by local chiefs. They were not about to allow a young foreigner to weaken their hold over local commoners, the king's lease-grant notwithstanding. By the end of the year, Hooper had made peace with the chiefs, hired natives, obtained tools, built a rudimentary mill with wooden rollers, and thatched huts for his workers, and planted a nursery of indigenous cane." (Sugar Islands*, p. 27.)

Still, by 1847 Koloa was bankrupt. In December, Dr. Robert W. Wood, a physician from Augusta, Maine, after settling in Honolulu in 1839 and establishing his practice, purchased Koloa for $17,500. Hiring sugar experts, he quickly modernized the plantation, selling it in 1872 at a handsome profit, along with other successful sugar investments.

Missionary and private physicians with a little Western medical training were active in other cane producing districts. Long accounts of grueling trips on foot or horseback to see patients, particularly on Hawaii, were common. But despite well-meaning efforts to provide health care to the entire Hawaiian population, little organized or competent technology was available. A feeble understanding of public health principles, use of archaic cupping, bleeding, calomel, castor oil and other purges, went little beyond the arts of the native practitioner. Other than a few simple surgical interventions for rich or poor alike, prayer and resignation to pain and death were one's lot far into the nineteenth century.

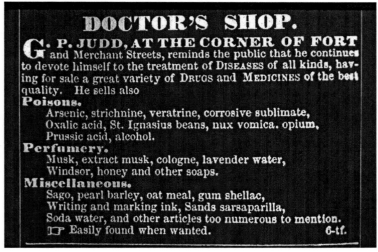

Doctors often supplied a remarkable range of sundries.

Not all of the scores of physicians whose lives touched early plantation life in Hawaii, were missionary-based. More secular interests brought scores of our early peers to practice in these challenging lands. In my own quiet tropical evenings, I often pondered the fragile threads of fate that tug at our lives, any one of which, when once spun, may shape an entire lifetime, or if broken, spawns quite another. And so with these early medical idealists and fortune hunters who cast their mid-Pacific lots, all had their personal threads for us to ponder along with our own.

CHAPTER 3

Threads of Fate

My own thread to a long happy life as a Hawaii physician on a tropical island must have begun as genetic. My ancestral family in Tyneside, England built ships; my childhood drawings, when the teacher passed out paper and crayons for "art class," were all of palm trees, islands and ships on deep blue seas, seeking sand and sun. I vaguely wanted to work in the warmth of cultural diversity, somewhere far away. After WW II service in Europe, further training, and a settled practice, my thread led me by one of fate's oddest detours to a Mount Baker, Washington ski lodge where I met an older doctor in wet snow up to the roof in the deep stillness of winter, with only the sound of a distant generator and no one around. We exchanged pleasantries. He had just left Honolulu to establish a practice in British Columbia because he had recently married an Alpine girl who hated Honolulu. For him it was—move or annulment. I listened to his story, which ended with "you'd love it in the islands." Wondering at the sanity of his new bride, I absent-mindedly pocketed a name he handed me, scribbled on an old envelope. The name was Dr. Nils Larsen, a medical giant in the islands.

Some months later, back at my pediatric practice in the cold and wet of Bellingham, Washington, I came across the name in a pocket of a pair of pants just back from the cleaner. My mostly forgotten, rediscovered ski lodge thread of fate led onward.

On a whim, I wrote Dr. Larsen a note. His reply:

"By Territorial Law, No openings in Hawaii without a Hawaii license preceded by one year of Hawaiian residency."

My potential Hawaii thread nearly snapped with the chilly thought, "I'd better put the chains on my tires on the way home so I can get up over the icy ramp into the garage."

One afternoon, more than a year later, the phone rang. It was the telephone company operator (we had them then). "Call for you, Doctor, from Hawaii." It was my Dr. Larsen. "Would you like to come to Hawaii? There is a plantation job open."

For a very long time I sat at my desk in a seething stew of euphoria, caution and fantasy, looking out at the mushy streets and cold Northwest drizzle, counting the big wet snowflakes sticking to the windowpane. Totally shocking my nurse who thought I had "lost it," I rearranged my appointments, caught a plane to Hawaii for a quick (one day) look, and grasped the thread to the rest of my life.

An opportunity that came with the Hawaiian offer, leading, in a way, even to this book, seemed as intriguing as the thought of living with warmth and adventure. In my 1950s fee-for-service practice, I saw the impending national disaster of uninsured care, and was intrigued by the chance to explore the freedom and benefits for patients and physicians alike, of fully prepaid care that was then a part of the wider social support of plantation life.

After six hectic weeks of moving furniture, cars, family, and dog, I had joined the legacy of plantation physicians in Hawaii, a whirlwind life change triggered many months before by a chance name scrawled on a grungy envelope. Unknown to me then, a parallel thread began long ago to wind slowly through the maze of Hawaiian history that shapes our island lives. As this thread was spun, tragic changes were coming to Kamehameha's tiny island kingdom.

HEALTHCARE HAWAII STYLE

Western Disease—Agent of Change in an Island Nation

Cook's arrival in 1778 brought the first serious biologic agents of change, syphilis and gonorrhea. Later, ships arrived with other new diseases such as cholera in 1804 that killed nearly 15,000, and with flu, mumps, pertussis, and especially measles that steadily took a steady, deadly toll. More subtly, traffic in alcohol and major lifestyle changes in diet and habit added to the carnage, but the most spectacular disaster was waiting for 1853 with a Hawaiian population already down from 140,000 to 80,000 in thirty years.

Smallpox—The Ship-borne Killer

The handful of physicians scattered around the islands from the time of the first missionaries in 1820 until the 1850s did what they could individually to provide care to an increasingly diverse population—Hawaiians, haoles, hundreds of sailors, immigrant producers of meat, hides, vegetables, and the early sugar planters—anyone who needed their rudimentary healing skills. Although new diseases that came by ship were severely decimating the Hawaiian people, medical care was not seen as a matter of public crisis. Contagion was not understood. Some public health concepts, although in place as quarantine laws as early as 600 A.D. in China and 1348 in Venice had not yet reached Hawaii.

The first contact with the outside world after hundreds of years of isolation brought fateful threads of contagion, snaring the native population of Hawaii in relentless coils of sickness, death and depopulation.

Apart from disease, alcohol, firearms, and emigration took their toll. By 1845, about 2000 Hawaiians were working on foreign vessels. Many chose never to return to the islands. Then, like a rogue wave in the midst of a hurricane, in mid-century the sad and steady destruction of the Hawaiian population peaked with a sudden epidemic.

Smallpox, a worldwide disease, had not yet appeared, but cases were reported in Hong Kong and Tahiti by the crew of the Don Quixote, which was probably "clean" by the time she reached Honolulu in 1841.

Efforts to vaccinate had been made in 1825 by a Honolulu physician, Dr. Abraham Blatcheley with an eighteen-month-old vaccine from London that was apparently inactive. It had long been known that contact with cowpox seemed to immunize milkmaids against smallpox—the ninth century Chinese were actually immunizing their patients. Although cowpox material was also being ordered from Boston, the long voyage around the Horn of the old, unrefrigerated vaccine in a zinc box probably was often found to be useless when administered, primarily to the missionaries and their children. Despite questionable vaccine supplies, by 1839, Dr. T. C. B. Rooke had vaccinated eight to ten thousand people, and in following years was assisted in his efforts by several other Hawaii physicians: Drs. G. Judd, D. Baldwin, G. Lathrop, and C. Wetmore.

Some physicians "inoculated" their patients—a different procedure, using lymph from active smallpox cases. Although this dangerous approach was often protective, it could easily kill, leading to some highly heated clinical disputes.

The epidemic of 1853, followed by efforts to repopulate the islands with productive workers, would change the nature of Hawaii's population forever.

CHAPTER 4

Thread of Death

The single most disastrous thread of fate, more accurately, a thick cable of woe that led to major depopulation of the islands and to the ultimate arrival here of most of us, was summarized in *Oahu's Ordeal, the Smallpox Epidemic of 1853*, by Richard A. Greer, published in a 1965 issue of the Hawaii Historical Review. These are some excerpts from his report:

The American ship, Charles Mallory, had arrived with a yellow flag flying from her foremast and a case of smallpox aboard. The harbor pilot, finding disease, left the ship outside and came back to report to the Board of Health. Dr. S. P. Ford, of Honolulu, then went out and saw the cook or steward "down with a clear case." A consultation of physicians decided that vaccinated passengers and the mailbags should land after bags and baggage had been fumigated. The ship anchored off Waikiki, and all six passengers, all vaccinated, came ashore. They took salt-water baths, had an entire change of clothes, and went into quarantine for two weeks at today's Kapiolani Park. The fumigated mail was re-sacked, and the old bag destroyed. Dr. Edward Hoffman took charge of the group at the park. The sick man was lodged in a grass house on a reef island surrounded by water at high tide, quarters offered by Prince Lot Kamehameha, where the man lived alone for five weeks. No one wanted to nurse him, but one member of the Board of Health went out daily to feed him.

The ship was quarantined for 14 days, fumigated, and brought into port. All clothing and bedding materials were burned. The ship left with the convalescent, whose grass house was also burned. The government had no money to pay quarantine expenses, so W. C. Parke, Marshal of the Kingdom, advanced $1,500 of his own (later repaid)."

Dr. Ford's report of smallpox on the Mallory caused a furor. For three days, doctors consulted with each other, nine in all, and the U.S. Consul. The Privy Council appointed Dr. Gerrit Judd to head the defense against the impending epidemic, offered thanks, invited anyone who might be useful—physicians, missionaries or others throughout the island—to donate their services, and pointed out that it could not provide for "any great expense," a delightfully modern political sentiment.

The leading newspaper of the day, *The Polynesian*, again called for stricter measures than those used for the *Mallory*, and urged immediate vaccination. An editorial in the *Weekly Argus* noted that because of the costs involved to send doctors out, vaccine should be supplied to the missionaries with a royal proclamation mandating vaccination despite its limited success.

Early in March 1853 missionary Richard Armstrong, the minister of public instruction, announced that he had "procured vaccine matter and distributed it to a good extent." Vaccination was going on among the islands. At about the same time the *Polynesian* remarked that both foreigners and Hawaiians were making much use of vaccine. Its story optimistically concluded: "with this and other precautions we trust we shall hear no more of a disease which justly excited considerable alarm when it was first announced among us."

Honolulu was calm while fate fashioned its final strand, the massive depopulation of villages, plantations, and even "urban" Honolulu. Although smallpox had been reported on board some weeks before in Australia, there was no stir when an American brig named *Zoe* arrived on 23 March 1853 or when she left two weeks later. On Friday the 13th of May (note the date), a man came to Marshal Parke's office telling of two "sick" at Maunakea Street. Parke went out and found smallpox. News was hurried to the Board of Health. Other cases soon surfaced, and as was earlier written, "so began *ke wa kapela*," the smallpox time—a time of massive death, incredibly deadly social destruction and grief.

Once again, to draw from Richard Greer's 1965 monograph containing a telling missionary letter. "The board of health is active and prompt. Vaccination is going on. Only one person in our family has been vaccinated with effect, though all have had it done repeatedly. We employ Dr. Hardy. The smallpox is increasing. We fear death will make sad havoc—you may hear that some of us have been hurried into eternity. May no one be called unprepared."

Now the smallpox began to eat its way, slowly at first, through the city. On 16 May, Kamehameha III approved "an act relating to the Public Health." It provided that the king with the consent of the Privy Council should appoint a commission of three people to act without pay and upon them should rest the duties intended and expressed in the act of 8 May 1851, setting up a board of health for the entire kingdom. Many other details followed, with the appointment of three health commissioners, G. P. Judd, T. C. B. Rooke, and W. C. Parke. Operating funds could be withdrawn from the public treasury. At the outset of the epidemic, a hospital had been fitted up at once, and sixteen sub-commissioners were appointed, many of them missionaries. Over the next few weeks, a flood of reports from Oahu and other islands numbered deaths in the hundreds. On 6 June, Judd told the Privy Council that the sickness was spreading fast and that "The people would not be confined and would not regard anything said to them."

At an emergency meeting of the Privy Council on 9 June, Armstrong introduced a resolution advising the king to order 14 June a day of "humiliation, fasting and prayer, that the Almighty may remove from among us the smallpox now spreading everywhere." The proclamation was approved.

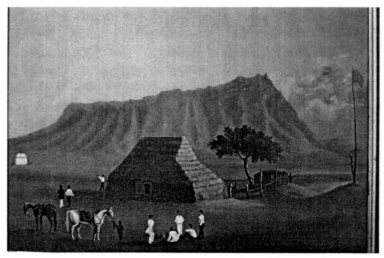

Smallpox quarantine station on site of present Kapiolani Park, Honolulu, HI. 1853 painting by Paul Emmert. Property of Mission House Museum, Honolulu, HI.

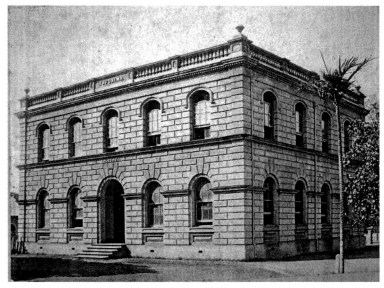

Honolulu Board of Health Building, 1884. The Department of Health was formed in 1859 by Kamehameha III.

The *Weekly Argus* editor found all this unworthy. "Preaching up national calamities as divine judgment to a people such as the Hawaiians who were of doubtful morality it tended to confirm a fatalism to which the people were already too prone. Shortcomings should not be excused by assigning a natural result to a supernatural cause." It was laudable touch of reason over superstition.

Mortality in some areas was approaching fifty percent. Burials were becoming a problem. Dr. William Hillebrand, of Honolulu who would later lead repopulation efforts by arranging immigration, noted the Hawaiian's habit of burying victims inside their houses or in the immediate vicinity, and wrote of a case in which the bodies of a man and child were thrown together in a low pit under the very mats where a number of people slept.

In these exhausting times, tempers flared. Three of the commission doctors signed a petition to fire Dr. Gerrit Judd from his post. Many people hid in the mountains to escape the police. Bodies were found unburied and partly eaten by dogs and hogs that roamed in and out of Hawaiian grass houses and prowled everywhere. Many corpses went to the grave without coffins. They were so lightly covered that animals rooted and scratched them up. Many said they were the chief spreaders of the disease. Doctors reported incredible misery everywhere. Bodies lay in mass graves all over Honolulu, complicating urban building even today as unidentified bones are unearthed. But not all was strife. Public subscription raised money to feed and nurse some of the sick who were in desperate need of help

As the crisis deepened, the *Weekly Argus* spread bitter comments. Wyllie's recommendations of 1844 for mass immunization had never been carried out, all being left to Providence or accident. Parke, the sheriff, and the doctors gave their service without exception, going anywhere they could, day or night, with advice, medicine, and cheering words, without pay or hope of any.

Richard Greer reports further that on 18 July 1853, Honolulu foreign residents, dismayed, called a public meeting at the courthouse leading to selection of a new committee of 12, plus all the Honolulu physicians, for new recommendations. This resulted in several sets of houses that became small hospitals, division of the islands into districts (20 on Oahu alone), and the start of a "vaccination hospital," actually more of a vaccination outpatient facility. The main line of battle was in the houses and huts of the stricken.

Doctors could not carry the load. Many victims were never

seen by a physician. It was common to find whole families sick, or to discover only dead bodies in a house. Carts to haul bodies were in short supply, as were gravediggers. The disease was decimating its labor supply. Four immune prisoners were released to dig graves and were later pardoned.

An account book in Hawaiian covering hospital operations for May and June shows a total expense of $483.52 for food, blankets, and mosquito nets. The hospital diet included beef, molasses, spices, poi, and rice. Despite offering the best nursing care in its day, it was almost impossible to convince patients to go there. The expectancy of death and vivid accounts of ghosts scattered terrified patients and the local populace to the very end of the scourge.

Where had the smallpox come from? It was a much-argued question, with no certain answer even today. Had it come from the Mallory? Thrum, an author who had been in Honolulu during the epidemic, and who later became well known for his annual *Thrum's Almanac of Hawaii*, wrote that public opinion laid the blame here. Sheriff Parke said the vessel could not have been guilty since "some months" had passed between her sailing and the outbreak, but there were rumors of possible contacts with the Mallory's single smallpox patient. The newspaper *Polynesian* finally reported (perhaps rightly) that the disease probably arrived in the 100 chests of old clothing brought from San Francisco and sold at auction in Honolulu.

Dr. Judd's wife agreed that the scourge was supposed to have come in the trunks of old clothes and that the first victims were two women who had washed some of the garments, but this was disputed by the dates of the first cases. Other stories prevailed, and other ships were blamed. No one knows the truth.

As the epidemic wound down, two concerns of the medical men of the day played across the scene. One was the dispute between those who believed in vaccination with cowpox that Edward Jenner had discovered in 1796 when he noted accidental immunity among his English milkmaids who had contracted cowpox from their animals.

Others, who rejected Jenner's sound discovery, advised inoculation with live smallpox vaccine from recovering patients, a very dangerous alternative to cowpox inoculation. Valid comparison of the success of these immunizations in Hawaii was undermined by the probable deterioration of much the vaccine shipped without refrigeration from a half a world away.

The second concern of the stressed Hawaiian government and local physicians was the question of payment of physicians and officials who felt they had valid claims on the government for services provided during the epidemic. The House of Nobles in 1855 had appointed two commissioners "to take evidence on all claims against the Government, on account of services rendered during the prevalence of the Smallpox, and give a report to the legislature in 1856."

As is likely in such claims, nothing happened. The 1856 legislature ignored the matter and indefinitely postponed the issue. In 1859 when it somehow became a matter of negotiation between the Hawaiian government and the United States, Parke, for his heroic efforts at the onset of the scourge, was granted $800 to recompense his own outlay for patient care. Dr. Hillebrand received a pittance, and the rest of the team, a comment of gratitude by the King on behalf of his subjects. How ironic, that despite the nearly 150 years and incredible economic development separating us from these events, we are still faced with insoluble problems of how to pay for health care. Critical medical efforts often go unpaid. It is a mark of the profession. Roughly fifteen thousand dead from smallpox was the final blow to Hawaii's native people after six decades of depopulation from syphilis gonorrhea, cholera, measles, influenza in 1826, social chaos and despair.

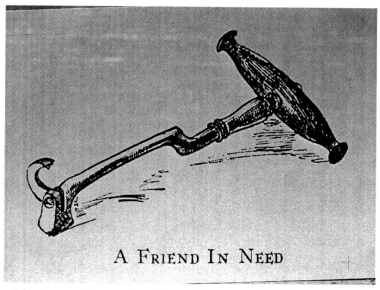

A FRIEND IN NEED

Advertisement for use of rotating tooth extractor, 1849. Anaesthetic was morphine, or whiskey, or nothing. Teeth were simply pried out by twisting the handle.

Sept 29, 1849.

DENTISTRY!

DR. COLBURN, DENTIST, from NEW YORK, would respectfully inform the citizens of Honolulu and the adjacent Islands, that he has opened his rooms over the old Polynesian Office, adjoining the residence of Capt. Snow, near the THEATRE, where he would be pleased to see those who may require his services.

TEETH EXTRACTED with the FORCEPS only.

☞The soreness removed from the most·sensitive Teeth, so as to be filled without pain or killing the nerve.

☞Families waited upon at their residences, if required. · [sep29tf20

Co-Partnership.

Itinerant and local dentists practiced in early Honolulu. Dental office and home services were available. Advertisements in The Polynesian, 1849.

NOTICE.

ON ACCOUNT OF THE LARGE INCREASE in the cost of Provisions, and the necessaries of life generally, the Board of Trustees of the Queen's Hospital, has decided to increase the rate for the maintenance and treatment at the Hospital of foreign patients to $1.50 per day, exclusive of expense incurred for wine and watchers, in special cases. This rate to commence from the 1st February. Per order.

794 4t   F. A. SCHAEFER, Sec'y.

Notice of rate increase after opening of the hospital.

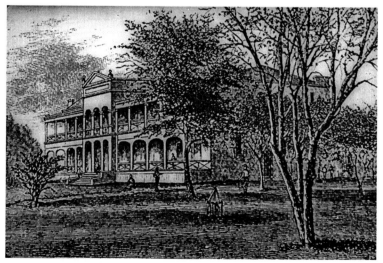

Queen's Hospital, Honolulu, after 1859, where plantation patients with complex problems were often sent.

Estimation of the population of the Hawaiian Islands during a little more than one hundred years of contact shows the effect on the indiginous Hawaiian population of Western disease and the lifestyle changes of the period.

Population of Hawai'i

Year	Total Population	Native Hawaiian Population
1778	250,000	250,000
1831-32	130,313	unknown
1853	73,137	71,019
1872	56,897	51,531
1890	89,990	40,622

Source: Nordyke, Eleanor C. The Peopling of Hawaii, Honolulu, Hawaii: University of Hawaii Press; 1989. Pg 174, 178.

From an estimated high of at least a quarter million Hawaiians living on the islands when Captain Cook arrived, the population fell in the ensuing century to less than ninety thousand, and of those remaining, only half were native Hawaiians. Native leaders, royalty, *alii*, missionary entrepreneurs and adventurers who had come to cast their lots for profitable island ventures, were suddenly faced in mid century with economic disaster. Major productivity was necessary to develop and sustain the government, and burgeoning business interests. Willing labor was missing. It was soon negotiated for by many, from kings on down through the commercial community.

In 1855, King Kamehameha IV summed up the situation for his legislature:

"The decrease of our population is a subject in comparison with which all others sink into insignificance."

CHAPTER 5

Repopulation—New Challenges for Hawaii's Medical Community

To rescue the mid-century economy, to support the rapidly changing lifestyle of the Islands, and particularly to develop sugar production, imported labor was the only solution. In 1850 the Royal Hawaiian Agricultural Society convened and passed the "Act for the Government of Masters and Servants" allowing imported labor. Captain John Cass, of the bark *Thetis*, was commissioned to bring a supply of laborers from China to work on the sugar plantations. He soon returned with 175 field hands and 20 domestic servants seeking a new life.

A few Chinese workers had already come to the islands, usually as ship's crew members, and stayed. Because they were found to be excellent employees, more were sought through formal arrangements made by government leaders and plantation owners. In their 2000 book, *Sugar Islands*, historian William H. Dorrance and sugar plantation industry expert Francis S. Morgan recount the booming success of these repopulation efforts and some of the problems encountered in adapting to the needs of the newcomers:

> *"Some five hundred Chinese were brought from Amoy province in 1852. They contracted for five years of labor in return for their transportation, housing, food, clothing, and pay of three dollars a month. Despite an initial period of turmoil, caused in part by the language barrier, and*

the choice of many to desert their plantations for a town-centered life of independent laborer or small scale shopkeeper, these Chinese were valuable employees. Few women were among them, and they lived in rudimentary barracks or bunkhouses that cost little to construct and maintain. The terms of their contracts largely held them to their assigned plantations under penalty of law for desertion or refusal to work."

All of these new, exotic groups were human beings needing health care in a clean, safe world. Most of the early immigrant groups came with individuals among them who professed some medical knowledge, and informally provided rudimentary care within their culture. It soon became clear to plantation owners that their future success lay in the health and well being of their laborers and their families, and that more sophisticated care was wanted. Licensed physicians were hired by companies and the Hawaiian government Adequate nutrition, clean, safe housing and maternal and child health programs were developed, as much to insure productivity as to quell disease. The generalist was the key physician until after WWII when further transportation of problem patients to specialists became feasible. Despite the cultural and language barriers, Hawaii's health steadily improved until it became a model of community and industrial health and welfare, only now threatened by the international lifestyle irrationalities that invite metabolic and degenerative disease. Dorrance and Morgan continue:

"The labor problem seemed to be solved. Unfortunately, the market for sugar had collapsed after California was admitted to the Union in 1850. Under the U.S. Tariff Act of 1846, a percent tax applied to sugar imports was now levied against Hawaiian sugar exported to California. As a result, numerous enterprises in Hawaii went bankrupt and importation of labor ceased, but when the

Civil War broke out in 1861, this created a windfall for Hawaii's sugar producers. Labor recruiters were sent to Hong Kong and other Chinese ports. In 1864, the Kingdom established a Bureau of Immigration to control the new flow of new workers.

In 1865 Chinese immigration to Hawaii was renewed. It continued for over four decades, until 1987, when 56,700 Chinese had arrived in Hawaii. Of these, some 8,000 arrived from California. United States exclusion laws prevented further arrivals after annexation in 1898.

Planners, noting the industry and dependability of Asian workers, decided to try employing Japanese. The Kingdom arranged with independent contractors to recruit in Japan for contract laborers. In 1868, when this began, rural Japan was suffering a depression and work in far away Hawaii was an appealing prospect. An initial shipment of some two hundred indentured Japanese arrived in Hawaii that same year followed by a 17-year hiatus caused by political difficulties and a recession in sugar."

Through contractual arrangements made with Portugal by Dr. William Hillebrand, a former member of King Kalakaua's Privy Council who traveled to the Madieras Islands in 1877, by 1896, seventeen-thousand five hundred Portuguese had emigrated to Hawaii, most with their wives and children, in stark contrast with the first Japanese arrivals who numbered 149 men and 6 women. The arrival of the Portuguese with their families set a new standard of need for housing, medical care, schooling and social organization which was slowly met. The expense of community improvement for these people was well rewarded by their work ethic and productivity, which soon led to their participation in middle plantation management.

Japanese immigration resumed after King Kalakaua's befriending the Emperor of Japan in 1881 during a world trip;

nearly sixty-nine thousand Japanese had come to Hawaii by 1897. Dorrance and Morgan spoke of the fate of indenture contracts, their demise with annexation, and the effect on housing and pay.

"*All ethnicities of workers often refused to renew their contracts. Many returned to their homelands, so replacements were continuously needed. Modern machinery, introduced in the 1850s and 1860s, speeded sugar production, creating demand for more acreage and field labor. As the plantations grew in size, they distributed laborers to strategically located villages called "camps." Each had assigned fields and was presided over by a foreman. As with mainland farms of the time, none of these early camps had electricity, running water, kitchens, sewage, or indoor toilets. Living conditions were primitive but far better than where the immigrants had come from.*

Northern Europeans and south sea islanders were hired around 1880, but they didn't work out. It was up to the Chinese, Japanese, Portuguese, and a few native Hawaiians to carry the Hawaii sugar industry into the twentieth century.

Annexation

Annexation notions were in the air in the late 1800s that were anticipated with mixed emotions by the planters. Some like Isenberg and Spreckels, German citizens, and Davies, a British national, none of whom were of missionary background, had supported the monarchy and resisted annexation. Other planters with New England roots who were more numerous, pressed for annexation by the United States. Following the Organic Act of 1900, which officially established annexation and ended labor contracts, workers saw themselves as being freed from their contractual agreements. In the next year, 22 strikes by Japanese and others occurred at various plantations They demanded better housing and higher pay. Agitators went to work in Honolulu and spread strike news to the plantation workers. The planters responded in 1907 by ending Japanese immi-

gration and bringing in workers from the Philippines which had been ceded to the United States by Spain in 1899 at the end of the Spanish-American war."

WILLIAM HILLEBRAND

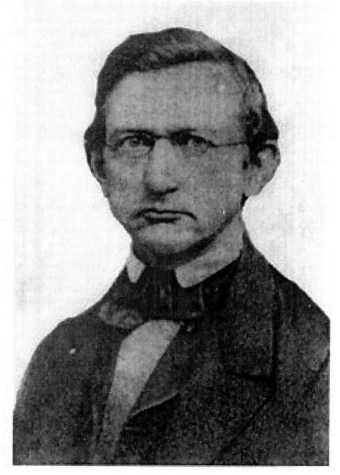

Dr. William Hillebrand

The Organic Act of 1900, while ending contract labor, made the citizens of Hawaii citizens of the United States, and subject to national statutes.

Passage of the Act complicated matters of Asian immigration, as Federal law prohibited Chinese emigration to any of the states or territories. Planters then focused on the U.S.-controlled Philippine Islands as a new source of workers who could enter Hawaii as nationals. In December 1906, Albert F. Judd, as an agent of H.S.P.A., brought three hundred Filipinos to Hawaii. By 1930, 100,000 had come to Hawaii, by 1946, another 6,000, and now a steady flow was the norm, but a working life on a plantation was no longer their destination, or the choice of the thousands of decendants of those workers who arrived during the early years of heavy migration.

Looking back, these were truly fruitful years. Beginning in sugar and pineapple plantation toil and deprivation, the relationships of managers with labor improved and the lot of workers grew as wealth was generated for everyone. Tough union demands over decades contributed to a humane, productive system which appeared reasonably stable into the nineteen seventies, only to be wiped out by lower costs of foreign production, and the lure of far more profitable land use in Hawaii than farming.

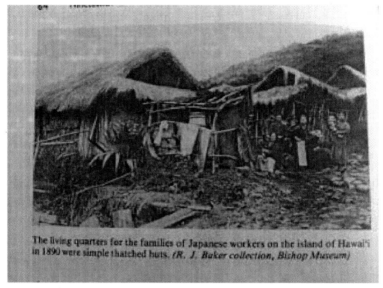

The living quarters for the families of Japanese workers on the island of Hawaiʻi in 1890 were simple thatched huts. *(R. J. Baker collection, Bishop Museum)*

An early substandard plantation camp, late 1800s. Bishop Museum Photo.

Today, the cost of our daily material wants—homes, transportation, tuition, services and entertainment, can no longer be met through the earning power of Hawaii's entire plantation world. But from that world, we have inherited a remarkably productive work ethic and the respect of management for labor, forged during recent years of relative amity. (True, there were early years of vicious labor-management strife that led up to the strikes of 1909 and 1920 in which twelve thousand strikers and their families were forced, at the heart of a flu epidemic, from their plantation homes within forty-eight hours, losing all pay, housing, and health care for six months).

Further strikes, almost annually, resulted in consolidation of union power that has spread from the plantations to the shipping and visitor industries to assure improved working conditions, wages and fringe benefits.

After 1920 the plantation companies began to realize the collective power of labor. Trustees of the Hawaii Sugar Planters' Association quietly increased wages by half, and began social welfare, housing, and recreational programs on the plantations. To insure healthful leisure- time activities, gymnasiums were built, competitive sports programs were launched, movie theaters were provided, and strong community life was encouraged.

As medical technology advanced, health care was seriously addressed, physicians were hired, and rural clinics and hospitals were built. Joint efforts of the plantation companies with those of the state and county governments spawned child and maternal health services. At the time I arrived in the 1950s, a unique plantation health care system was in place, born of a comfortably non-combustible mixture of union pressure, company enlightened self-interest, and technical innovation. With excellent housing, sanitation and water supplies came fully funded "cradle to grave" medical care. Workers and families thrived in the effective health care system that lasted until the recent years of plantation closures.

It was a rough voyage of social advance from the brutal working conditions of pre-WWI plantation life to the relative comfort and security of its closing years. Enormous change came from new concern with the wellbeing of workers; including the development of county and state clinic services, and on-site physician and nursing care in plantation and government hospitals.

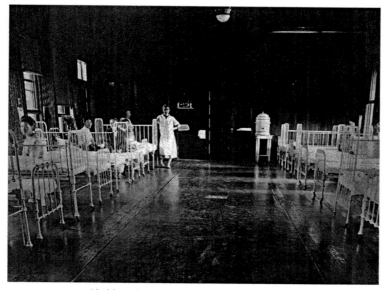

Childrens' Ward, Puunene Hospital, 1924.

Unions, plantation companies, public health workers, and the physicians, each with shared community interests, made it all work. Central governance of the system by the plantation companies, backed by our extensive Public Health Nursing system and rural hospital network, were for Hawaii, the magic mix. Despite time and plantation demise, we still live with very few payers, which simplifies coverage here. Nationally, we need to launch a similar universal health system with perhaps one or two payers, preferably one, with strong Federal or State public health program support of community care centers, clinics, and hospitals. To do this will take political guts and a violently aroused public.

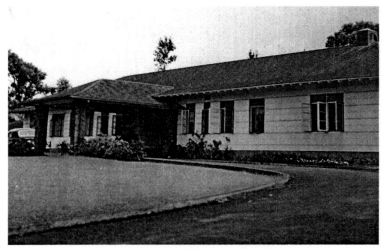

Laupahoehoe Plantation Hospital, 1924.

CHAPTER 6

Some Plantation Labor Stories

On one dreamy Sunday afternoon in my new home in Kohala, possibly one of the most beautiful spots in the vast Pacific, I was watching some gathering storm clouds that boded no good, when a boy on horseback rode up to say that a man had fallen from his horse, and was lying unconscious in his pasture. Indeed he was, with clear signs of a badly injured head.

With help, we soon had him in the hospital, but by then things began to fall apart. Here again, fate was spinning sundry threads, one celebrating Murphy's third law: *anything that can go wrong will.* We now had the howling wind and horizontal rain only the tropics can muster, washing out any plans for transportation. At least the power was still on.

A skull x-ray was not helpful, and our patient was slowly getting more and more distant. The nearest neurosurgeon was in Honolulu, and in any case, moving the man was out of the question. The storm-downed trees on the only route to Hilo and rudimentary airports many miles away were against us. Should we call Honolulu anyway?

Fortunately, the phone worked, the surgeon was there, and without hesitation, he told me the man most likely was bleeding beneath his skull, a condition that required draining, and soon. This involved having to make a small hole in the skull above the site where we thought the problem might be, and opening the dura, covering of the brain, to release the collected blood—so far so good. Looking through our instrument collection, there was nothing to make the "burr hole" needed to get at the bleed. We had read or heard somewhere that this problem had been met before with ordinary carpenters' tools.

Lady Luck was with us. We were on a practically self-sufficient plantation with old-school artisans (usually older Japanese gentlemen with exotic tools who could make anything). We had a machine shop, plumbing shop, electrical shop, and happily, an open carpenter shop. There, hanging on the wall was a perfect right- sized ball shaped countersink bit that would work, and the brace to use it. Back in the hospital, we boiled the whole works in hot water, opened the skull (admittedly a long shot just where to bore), nicked the dura, and the fluid came out. Our patient survived, recovered consciousness, and with proper attention, was soon out of the hospital.

Slowly, during the first months of melding my mainland cultural background with the bucolic routine of plantation life, I began to see deep differences between my own demeanor and that of new local friends, neighbors, and patients—touches of laconic acceptance of the full range of life's vicissitudes, from waiting weeks for a Sears Roebuck package to stoic patience in a long illness or in the actual face of death. A pervasive philosophy of "no big thing" and "whatever" was heard everywhere as "no beeg ting" and "whateva." Asian equanimity rooted in Buddhism softened confrontation, and most issues were resolved with respect and humor—a subtle facet of island life.

In 1957 during a strike against Kohala Plantation where I worked, the workers asked the mainland-born manager if they could use the plantation's heavy equipment and have a supply of fuel and materials to build a children's wading pool in a windward cove. The answer was yes, as a matter of course, and work proceeded.

In the later years of the plantations, labor relations at this level of accommodation between labor and management were common. Among plantation managers there was generally a good-faith intent to improve the lives of workers.

The ILWU, the International Long Shore and Warehouse Union, was respected and after 1943 became the ruling voice of Hawaii workers, resulting in a sharp upgrade in the quality of plantation life. Today the ILWU has 22,000 island members working in many industries.

On one occasion, one of the plantation workers, an ILWU field hand representative about my size had to go to the mainland for a union meeting. My recent arrival in Kohala from the mainland suggested that I might own a suit, which he did not. He and his wife came over one evening and after amiable introductions, they tentatively inquired about the possibility of borrowing said suit. It fit perfectly. Suitably attired, he went to his meeting The suit came back nicely cleaned and pressed, but I cannot recall ever wearing it again in Hawaii's sartorial utopia where wearing a suit often arouses suspicion along the lines of "who is this guy and what is he trying to sell?" Cooperative relationships, large and small were the daily flow of plantation life, perhaps as an endorphic response to the beauty and peace of waving cane and the magic of perfectly temperate days and nights.

It was not always thus. In his 1984 book, *Pau Hana*, University of California professor Ronald Takaki wrote of the frequent and vicious early strikes beginning as early as 1841 on Kauai Island's Koloa Plantation with a demand for a wage increase from 12.5 cents to 25 cents a day. The strike was broken in two weeks. In 1881, forty-two Norwegian workers at the Alexander and Baldwin Plantation on Maui struck because of poor food. Eighteen went to jail with harsh sentences and were driven on foot 16 miles to their confinement by two mounted officers with revolvers and a whip. At Kohala Plantation on Hawaii in 1891, two hundred Chinese workers felt they were being cheated on their pay and refused to work until it was resolved. Management collected a body of men and rode through the group with bullock whips. Government officers jailed 55 of the strikers in leper cells.

Takaki states further that "on Ohahu in 1894 on Kahuku plantation, Japanese contract laborers had been abused by the overseers. Two hundred workers walked 38 miles over the tortuous Pali Road to Honolulu to protest to the local Japanese official, Goro Narita, the Japanese Charge d'Affaires to the Hawaiian Republic. Arrested by police and fined $5 each, the strikers were forced to walk back to Kahuku, their grievances ignored by the government. After the Organic Act took effect in 1900 freeing workers from their contracts, strikes multiplied and management found itself in a new world."

One Maui manager, at the time, warned the Hawaii Sugar Planters' Association trustees that big trouble lay ahead, and he was right. Japanese laborers on the Sprecklesville Plantation struck to end all contracts. Swinging clubs and throwing stones, 200 strikers fought a posse of 60 policemen and overseers armed with black snake whips. Although beaten and forced to retreat to their camps, the workers won the strike and contracts ended.

Again, in 1909, a major uprising, primarily by Japanese workers over the issue of higher pay and equal pay for the various ethnic groups doing the same work, led to a four-month battle. The prolonged conflict led to 5000 workers from surrounding plantations invading the city of Honolulu and sheltering in theatres, storefronts, and vacant buildings. A Palama kitchen served three meals a day to over 2,200 people. The Physicians Association, a group of Japanese doctors, provided medical care, and many organizations contributed funds, as did sympathetic plantation workers on other islands.

Further strikes have occurred since the turbulent times in the first part of the twentieth century, but they have been relatively benign, lacking the early year violence and mass movement into the streets and parks of angry desperate people. After years of strife to reach power equity, labor-management communication is better tuned to avert disaster.

The vicious exploitation of early plantation workers is deplorable. Many heroic people changed it, and now, in our media and small talk, we find real nostalgia for many of the positive values of recent plantation life. And indeed, in later years it was in many ways a good life, freed of hard labor by marvelous machines, made safe and comfortable by great gains in housing, wages, and cradle-to-grave health care, and the emergence of a unique ethnic amity.

As plantations sold houses and land to workers for token sums, increasing wages and more leisure time brought beautification of residential areas, community pride, and a wide sense of racial and social equality.

State Representative Michael Y. Magaoay, recalls his youth in the hill camp of Waialua Sugar Plantation in the nineteen fifties and sixties. Here are some of his recollections:

"It was in the plantation camps that so many of Hawaiian cultural traditions were preserved, shared, and passed on through the generations. Kinship existed between the cultural groups, with mothers watching over all the kids, no matter what camp they belonged to- and over the many single men...People helped each other without being asked. Meals were always shared...though no one had much money, toys and gifts were handmade and exchanged from the heart. People trusted each other. There was mutual respect for how hard everyone worked for what they had, and for the homes and possessions of others, so no one saw the need to lock their doors. Many of the values of this way of life in plantation communities are still alive today. In1990 when my son was born, I moved my family back to Waialua because I wanted them to experience a way of

life. . .that we would never see in Hawaii again. . .kinship, trust, ethnic tolerance and appreciation; values that were forged in the sugar and pineapple plantation camps." (*Honolulu Advertiser,* 5 Feb 2006).

The loss to the Islands of plantation life occurred not because of a change in work ethic or culture of workers. It was the lure of wild offshore profits made possible through the growing of sugar and pineapples in third world countries, and the boom in land values that scotched the possibility of Hawaiian sugar cane and pineapple any longer supporting our United States mainland life style to which we have all become accustomed.

Although the plantations are all but gone, a critical legacy remains- the comforting aura of being "local" which usually means a plantation background, recent or past, of place and family, imbued with a set of mores that warms our interracial relationships. It is a culture built on the concept of *ohana* or extended family, a powerful "one for all" idea. In Hawaii this "equal sharing" idea has actually reached into the social concept of universal access to health care, provided here today at a level rare in mainland states. Hawaii's remarkably generous health services have grown out of decades of government supported physician care and Public Health efforts launched by Kamehameha III, supported by generations of physicians, cooperative plantation managers and their companies. How did we arrive at this unusual point in our medical and social history?

The next chapters, drawn from eye-witness accounts of earlier times bring nostalgia, amusement, and respect for how successfully health care coverage has developed in Hawaii. Major challenges arise such as Medicare cuts and scarcity of specialists, and the overwhelming problem of care access in mainland states.

NILS PAUL LARSEN

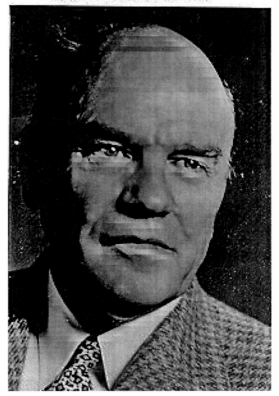

Dr. Nils P. Larsen, from 1922 through 1964, was a powerful force
in medicine and public health in Hawaii, holding many hospital and
government positions in industrial and plantation medicine, founding the
Territorial Plantation Physicians' Association in 1944.

CHAPTER 7

View from 1956

In 1856 King Kamehameha IV and Drs. Robert Wood and William Hillebrand launched Hawaii's first medical society. A hundred years later Dr. Nils Larsen, Hawaii Medical Association President and Medical Advisor to the Hawaii Sugar Planters' Association, reviewed the plantation life style and health care practices of that historic time in the *Hawaii Medical Journal.* Excerpts from Dr.Larsen's accounts of the era contrast starkly with the conditions and practices I encountered on the plantations upon my arrival in 1956.

In 1882 the earliest description of plantation medicine in practice came from a Chinese laborer who arrived in that year.

According to Dr. Larsen, *"the labororer's first impression of the plantation camp was 'very sad'. Where he had expected to see a roomy place, he found himself in a crowded camp house. They slept in double-decker beds, 24 to each room. The meals, however, were very good, and they had pork about once a week. They worked from 6 a.m. to 5 p.m. Wages for the contract men (three years) were $12 a month. Since our hero had experience with oxen and plows in China, he received a dollar a day."* (Hawaii Medical Journal, March 1956, p. 325).

How the plantation world had changed by 1956! I then found happy workers, well paid, living productive lives in safe comfortable houses, free to seek opportunity wherever they wished. I soon discovered that these benefits had come, however, only slowly over many years.

Dr. Larsen continued:

"After working 12 years in Hawaii, our hero accumulated enough money to send for a picture bride from his boyhood village in China. He had his picture taken in Honokaa and sent this to the girl's family, whom he had written to ask if they had a single girl. He received in return her picture and, the hope that she might come. The reply being favorable, he made arrangements with the immigration office regarding his bride-to-be who had been a little girl when he left China. In due time she arrived and was admitted. She was sent to Honokaa and there became his wife.

In their little two-room house, which was all they were permitted in the early days, 12 children were born without a doctor in attendance. The husbands always helped at the births, and three days later they went to the plantation doctor to report the birth and get a certificate. It was considered a great shame to have a doctor at the time of birth. Also, the plantation doctor lived far away and never came to the people's homes." (*Hawaii Medical Journal*, March 1956, p.325).

By 1956 almost all deliveries were in hospitals, by a physician. In earlier times it was, among the Chinese and Japanese women, simply a matter of pride to give birth with only family assistance. Dr. Larsen's informant remembered boils, measles, smallpox and influenza, but no doctor. Hospitals came later, around 1900, usually small, located next to the plantation manager's office, attended by a "Government Physician," paid by the Territory and several adjacent plantations. Conditions were very much better in Hawaii for Dr. Larsen's plantation hand than they would ever have been in China—the worker never had any regrets about moving here; it gave his eleven children a better chance than they would have had in China. Most became happy teachers and business men, with comfortable homes and thriving families.

In 1888, Dr. Luis Alvarez who was born in Spain came as a doctor to Hawaii. He lived at Waialua and was the only physician from Kaena Point to Kaneohe. Medical practices of the day were primitive. Dr. Alvarez operated on patients who were lying on the kitchen table. The local minister was drafted to give the anesthesia. At that time, if a patient was so sick he could not be taken care of in his home, a plantation cottage was used to house him.

The first hospitals on the outer Hawaiian islands were built in the early 1900s on Maui at Puunene, at Lihue on Kauai, and on Hawaii the Pepeekeo Hospital was opened in 1910. Dr. Fred Irwin, who came to Hawaii in 1903 from McGill University and New York, reported the following:

> None of the six plantations in my area had a hospital. The same was true of every other plantation and political district on the Island of Hawaii up to as far as I can remember until about 1910, when a hospital was built at Pepeekeo for three plantations, Honomu, Pepeekeo and Onomea. Traumatic surgery was taken care of almost where it happened—such as the amputation of both hands that were crushed in the mill rollers. The anesthetist was the plantation bookkeeper, the operating table a door taken from the patient's quarters. In Hilo there was a building called a hospital that had been an ordinary house; there were a few patients, but it hardly deserved the name of hospital. (Hawaii Medical Journal, March 1956, p. 326).

The primitive facilities of these times with deplorable water and sewage systems spawned serious outbreaks of intestinal diseases. Dr. Irwin further wrote that:

> "At Puna, there was a crude twenty-bed hospital where one could do fairly clean emergency surgery. However there was not a mosquito screen on one window in this hospital, the beds were all made of wood, and the mattresses were stuffed with hay brought up from the stables in bales. With no plumbing of any sort, the place used privy vaults. These teemed

with flies that spread infection to the roofs from which it was washed by rain into the water tanks. Typhoid fever was running wild at this time, in 1906 and 1907. In a period of four months, shortly after coming to the district, 108 cases of typhoid fever were cared for in this so-called hospital, with one orderly and two maids, and an occasional helper from the family involved." (*Hawaii Medical Journal*, March 1956, p. 326).

In contrast, by 1956, I found that through excellent sanitation and widespread immunization, typhoid and cholera had been virtually wiped out. However, heavy infestations of roundworms, tapeworms, and other gastrointestinal parasites were common in Filipino newcomers.

Surgery facilities I found in 1956 Kohala, simple as they were in an old frame building with a leaky roof, were "Mayo Clinic" compared with what Dr. L.L. Sexton described as the environment for his surgery practice on Hawaii in 1909:

Operation—a must. How? Easy. A five gallon oil can, build a fire; instruments sterilized. Local preparation—soap and water—old rags soaked in strong Lysol as drapes. Anesthetic-chloroform—easy to carry. Anesthetist—mamasan, (any elderly bright Japanese lady) trained on the spot by hand signals. There is nothing new in the world. We practiced early ambulation in those days. Manual extraction of a retained placenta, with the patient's temperature 103 was not considered a problem. 'Hoe hana hana' (field work) the next day was routine for the new mother, bowing and hissing her thanks as I passed by. Not my skill, but the grace of God." (*Plantation Health* 13:13 July 1949)."

By 1956 obstetric practice had become safe in the plantation hospitals, and was universally expected by workers' families. At the request of the mothers, most of our deliveries in Kohala were done without anesthetics, and with minimal sedation. Deliveries were remarkably silent.

Dr. Thoms Keay, who came to Pepeekeo on Hawaii Island in 1921, said that during his first year in the district sixty- two babies died. Epidemics of typhoid and diphtheria were a yearly occurrence. Many Filipinos were victims of sudden death from beriberi, probably accounting for occasional "mystery deaths" before vitamin B-1 was understood. Swollen legs and failing vision, caused by beriberi, were everyday complaints.

One reason for the dramatic improvement in the health of plantation workers I encountered upon arriving in the late 1950s was the series of sanitation improvements in plantation communities made in the twenties and thirties. The program was the most comprehensive welfare drive in Hawaii history.

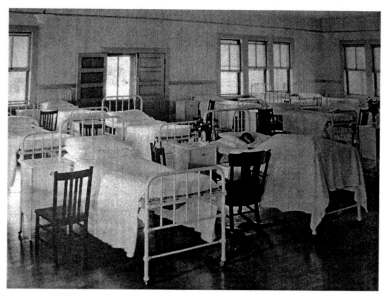

Mahulani Hospital, 1924.

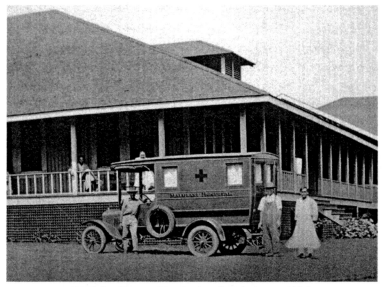

Wailuku County Hospital and ambulance, 1924.

In 1923, when 366 Filipino infants died in Hawaii, mostly on plantations, clearly something had to be done. Under the Territorial Board of Health a dairy campaign was started which resulted two years later in safe milk for Hawaii, and "healthy baby" clinics were set up across the Territory. The Queen's Hospital Research Department set up an experimental Health Center on Ewa Plantation under Dr. Nils Larson as Hawaii Sugar Planters' Association Medical Director. Its successful feeding clinic functioned for over twenty years. Industrialists became very health conscious and in 1930, the Hawaii Sugar Planters' Association appointed Dr. Nils Larsen as Medical Advisor.

A few of the Ewa Health Center's 1930 goals were to:
- Improve the general health of the plantation population and study the methods of bringing this about.
- Develop an experimental health center for all plantations,

from which health information and new evidence could be extended to all plantation doctors and staff through on-site instruction and regular publications.

- Conduct a thorough annual dental, laboratory and physical examination to discover other causes of ill health among plantation children.

H.S.P.A Health Bulletin, Aug. 46 #240

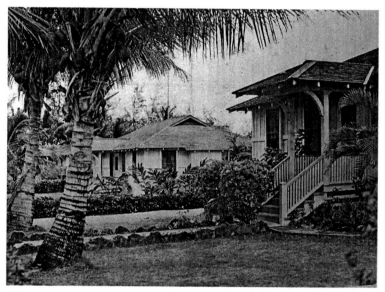

Plantation employee housing. Buildings and land were sold to workers for a token sum and moved to new sites on main roads with sewer lines, water and power supplies to encourage home ownership and community stability.

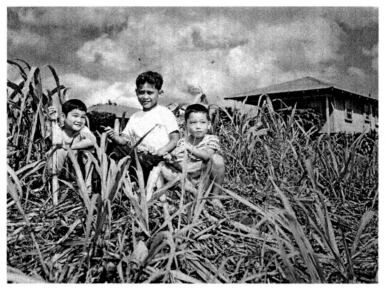

Workers' children playing in cane near plantation housing, Olaa, Hawaii, 1924.

A $3,000,000 improvement program affecting 5,000 employees and their families and plantations throughout the territory was undertaken by the HSPA in the 1930s. Homes were modernized, sanitation improved, and experimental health centers established. Modern gymnasiums and equipment for field sports in the community were provided for the 39 member plantations.

Results of the medical innovations centered at Ewa Plantation Hospital on Oahu vastly improved the entire plantation medical system. Firm statistical information on disease and accident incidence was gathered monthly, and health education spread to even the most distant communities through the plantation nurses, physicians, and *Plantation Health*, a quarterly journal, started in 1936. New medications, immunizations, and nutritional programs dramatically reduced mortality rates. Malnutrition, pneumonias, osteomylitis and tuberculosis faded with dietary changes and antibiotics. Penicillin, even before it was available commercially, was cultured and extracted by the Hawaii Sugar Planters' Association for use by plantation doctors.

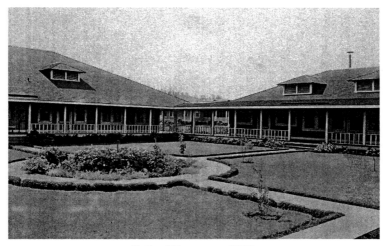

Kailua Dispensary, 1930.

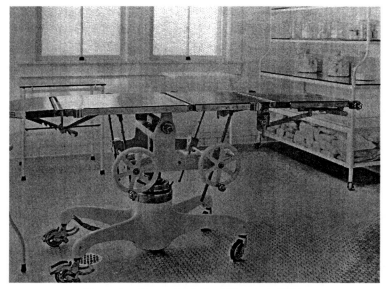

Operating Room, Mahulani Hospital, 1924.

Automobiles, plantation buses, and good roads brought patients to hospitals and clinics held in schools, gymnasiums, and church halls. A typical program I recall was a monthly "baby clinic" I held in the tiny settlement of Niulii in Kohala, Hawaii. There on the lanai of a small building next to an incredibly beautiful spread of plumeria trees overlooking the blue sea and Maui were happy mothers and children, awaiting their visits with the public health nurse and doctor. All were getting state of the art care in the most remote of rural settings, surely a triumph of organization and intent. And even the neighborhood dogs seemed pleased by the afternoon's activities, sniffing diaper bags and stroller wheels as they pondered the busy scene.

In such remote practice settings, physician "burn-out" from isolation was a risk. By the 1950s this was met by having two or more physicians available in most districts, allowing one to comfortably leave the area. Our leisure hours were greatly improved in the early sixties by the advent of continuous CB radio contact with the hospital from anywhere in the area from the mountains to the beaches. Such little things truly enhanced our rural lives.

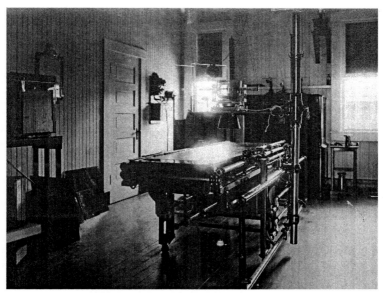

Xray table, Mahulani Hospital, 1924.

Another improvement in plantation care after WWII was the widespread use of specialist consultants throughout the islands. All known tuberculosis cases and their X-rays were reviewed periodically. A psychiatrist saw mental cases. Orthopedic consultants saw all cases for the Crippled Children's' Service as necessary. For many years, as a Pediatric Consultant for the Territory and then the State, I saw pediatric cases in Kona and Hilo. The Public Health Nurses and referring physicians in their districts meticulously prepared the patients and their problems for my visits. Further referrals of these children for further care in Honolulu were common, all at state or plantation expense.

The critical role of the plantation hospital in delivery of other than inpatient services was evident in the account by Dr. H. Paul Liljestrand, an Oahu physician active in the nineteen forties, when Aiea Hospital, together with its parent plantation closed with only a few days notice. With the sudden closure, he said, *Gone were the plantation clinics, the field nurse with her follow-ups, health surveys, health education, and regular physical examinations. A third of the men went to work for the neighboring plantation and thus continued to come under plantation medicine; for the remainder systematic medical care vanished overnight. Health service had disintegrated; diabetics had no insulin or urinalyses. Syphilis patients discontinued treatment because no camp nurse reminded them of its need. Although the hospital reopened as a private entity, long-term patients and even acute cases stayed at home; lack of an organized medical system with funding and access temporarily took its toll.*

Between the early 1900s and 1956 medical care improved dramatically in Hawaii. Our eyes glaze over on encountering statistics, yet we should note that by 1956, Hawaii's infant and maternal mortality had reached 10 and 0 per 100,000 of the population. No infants died of diarrhea or beriberi. Cases of tuberculosis had declined remarkably. There were no post-operative deaths reported from surgery, and venereal disease had become rare. After 1956, until the final demise of the plantation health care systems, monthly medical data flowed into management offices or was garnered by insurers or the state, as the Hawaii Medical Service Association (HMSA) became involved in coverage plans, so that today there exists a remarkably continuous record of changing disease patterns over the years, still useful for infectious disease and longevity studies for which data exist even into the late 1800s.

HEALTHCARE HAWAII STYLE

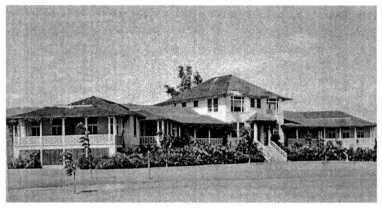

Ewa Hospital, 1936, containing new experimental clinical medical center, nutrition programs, Maternal and Child health care, TB and industrial health facilities.

Dr. Nils Larsen's view in 1956, and that of mainland consultants queried at the time, was that Hawaii had one of the best health systems anywhere in the country. While adequate nutrition in rural settings with easy ocean access for fishing, small gardens with plenty of fruits and vegetables, sanitation, and a stable community life were important in earlier times, additional amenities—the hard-won union realities of adequate pay and full-access to medical care—were critical as life changed to a more industrial life style. Improved sanitation through safe water supplies, sewage systems, adequate housing, and the rise of excellent nutrition were as important as full access to good health care. Although rapid changes after the 1950s, with major population influx, urbanization, developer's schemes and plantation closures have changed many lives, our state still leads the country in universally available health care. Hawaii's public health expenditures as reported for 2003 by the United Health Foundation led the nation at $499 per capita, remarkable in view of its small tax base. For comparison, below is a sampling of some other state public health expenditures, according to the United Health Foundation, a non-profit organization partnering with the Centers for Disease Control and the National Health Council.

State	Expenditure (2003)	Rank
Hawaii	$499	1
Alaska	$482	2
Wyoming	$354	3
New York	$316	4
Montana	$293	5
Idaho	$70	48
Arkansas	$64	49

http://unitedhealthfoundation.org

These are the amounts per person that were spent on public or population health for one year, in broad health care activities, excluding Medicaid reimbursement. They include direct health care services such as local health clinics, immunizations, cancer and tuberculosis screening programs, and population health expenditures such as infectious disease control, lab services, food safety, data collection, and a myriad of other services necessary to a modern community, as well as direct patient care for the indigent.

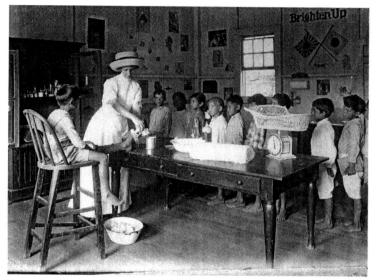

Health Clinic."Miss Saunders with children." 1930.

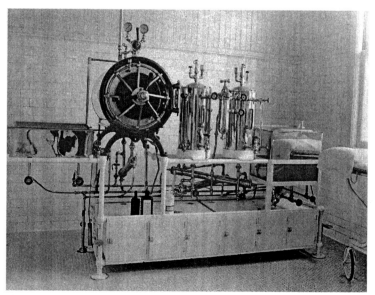

Steam Sterilizer, Mahulani Hospital, 1924

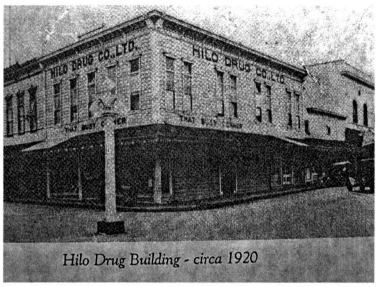

Hilo Drug Building - circa 1920

Hilo Drug Building in 1920. As roads improved, druggists often circuit-rode to plantations to supply dispensaries and hospitals.

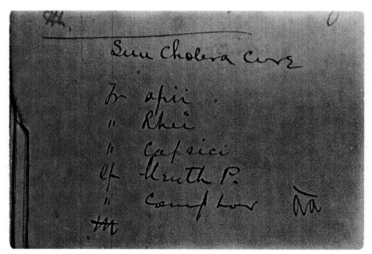

Cholera prescription, written in 1889 by Dr. Robert Williams.

CHAPTER 8

The Growth of Public Health, Housing, and Prosperity

Soon after I had become a small part of this remarkable rural medical system of the 1950s, I often wondered at the success of the organization, payment provisions, and clinical effectiveness of my predecessors, not only in our little world of Kohala, but wherever my travels in the islands led. Little did I then realize the jagged history of management/worker strife that slowly led, after annexation of Hawaii as a Territory of the United States 1898 to the "second revolution" of post WWII, spearheaded by the ILWU, and the powerful political ascendancy of many of the children of plantation workers to the highest places in island government.

One memorable evening, a distinguished visitor from Honolulu to our hospital in Kohala, opened for me one of the doors into Hawaii's social history. It was Dr. Richard K. C. Lee, President of the Hawaii Board of Health, a physician, and Doctor of Public Health, the head of the State Department of Health. The grandson of an early Chinese laborer, Dr. Lee was a consultant to the UN and held many health offices in the state government and in Pacific Rim countries. After describing his role in the state's brilliant public health history, he casually mentioned that his grandfather had been horsewhipped by a local plantation overseer when too sick to work. During the formative years of

Hawaii's Health Department, Dr. Lee's leadership in legislation addressed problem after problem. His influence enhanced programs tackling Hansen's Disease, tuberculosis, common childhood diseases, venereal diseases, milk- borne infections, mosquito control, nutrition, and immunization. All were successful public health efforts shared by the plantation companies and the Territory.

Clearly Dr. Lee was a paragon of competence and accomplishment. My appreciation of his rise from a family of field workers to international fame marked that evening, and our quiet talk answered the many questions I had about how he and so many other civic leaders had transcended the rigid barriers of the earlier plantation culture, leading it and Hawaii into our modern equitably multicultural society.

Early medical services to outer islands were provided by "traveling government physicians," funded by the Territorial Board of Health. Recommendations included that "they be furnished with medicine for the needy and with sufficient subsidies to enable them to maintain offices in sparsely settled districts in order to reach all the people living there." In 1901 these physicians were given the responsibility for registering births, deaths, marriages, and performing post mortems. Two years later, funds for these physicians were inexplicably cancelled and not restored for seven years. However, government-paid physicians, numbering 38 by the mid 1900s were again made the backbone of indigent care throughout the islands; many of these were also plantation physicians, paid by plantation companies. Their practices included private-pay patients from surrounding areas, such as Coast Guard personnel, teachers, and nearby ranch workers, whose care was paid for by contract with the ranch owners.

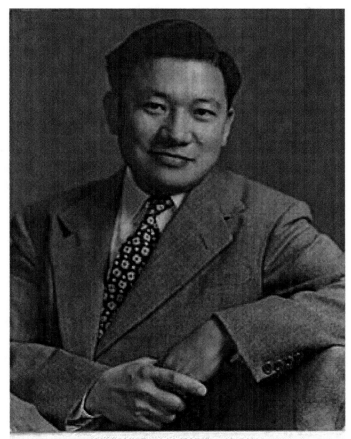

RICHARD KUI CHI LEE

Richard K. C. Lee, M. D. M. P. H. Internationally noted public health consultant to National Institute of Health, U. N., and W. H. O., and first Dean of the University of Hawaii School of Public Health.

In mid-century rural settings these "County" or "District" physicians still played many odd roles besides taking care of patients. On one occasion, for example, as Kohala District County Physician, I was presented by the police with a box of rather large bones that a local road crew had found in a bank alongside the roadway. Were they human bones, recent or old, and if so, what to do with them? Were they remains of a crime, or a peaceful burial? The problem was quickly solved. They were dog bones. That some had been thoroughly scraped, and many were missing suggested some happy culinary event.

Contract workers arriving in the late 1800s, quickly began to understand the opportunities open to them through hard work and wise investment. Freed by the provisions of annexation, which ended their indentured status in 1898, many of the workers, at great risk, branched out into highly profitable private endeavors. For many, plantation life was simply a stepping-stone to a better life.

As early as 1859, Honolulu's major newspaper, *The Polynesian*, ran an article about the rush of Hawaii's Chinese plantation workers moving to Honolulu. By 1882 only one third of the Chinese population of fifteen thousand still worked on plantations; and between 1887 and 1902, four thousand more Chinese left the sugar industry, while thousands more from all the racial groups left Hawaii for the West Coast. Between 1905 and 1907, one thousand Korean laborers left for California. By 1907, forty thousand Japanese had joined the mainland exodus. Money inducements and improved plantation living conditions helped stem the outflow, but finally, it required, through planter pressure in 1907, a federal order by Theodore Roosevelt to block Japanese and Korean emigration to the mainland.

Many years of bloody struggle for reasonable earnings and better living conditions lay ahead. In 1908, Oahu Japanese plantation workers formed a Higher Wages Association and went on strike in 1909. Strikebreakers were brought in at $1.50 a day—standard pay was $1.00. Leaders were jailed and fined. New strikes came in 1920. The attitude of these strikers contrasted with that of 1909 when workers in a letter to management expressed their "fondest and most cherished hope" that they might "continue to help the development and progress of your plantation" saying too, "it has become our painful burden to hereby respectfully present to you our request for reasonable increase of wages." The letter was ignored.

In the 1920 strike, bitter invective spewed from planters, labor leaders, and local publications. Some accommodations were made; but again in 1924, a Kauai strike of Filipinos resulted in twenty deaths, and the calling out of the National Guard. Strikes were not immediately successful, but owners clearly heard the message. Other deaths and injuries occurred, with one killed and two wounded at Lahaina, Maui, in 1905, and fifty workers injured in the "Hilo massacre" of 1938.

In response to these sporadic labor uprisings, modern, sanitized, healthcare-conscious plantation communities with good water supplies were launched in an unmistakable mix of paternalism and economic self-interest, despite the mounting expense of these improvements. Remodeling and new housing construction in the nineteen twenties cost millions of dollars. Single-family units were built, with a washhouse, bath, and outhouse. Running water, sewers, paving and lights lay far in the future, but these early amenities were appreciated and labor was appeased for the moment.

More improvements began in the 1930s adding larger houses with running water, sewer systems and inside baths. Newer plantations like Ewa on Oahu concentrated camp living by grouping their workers in houses near the mill, and transporting them to and from the fields on the plantation railroad.

As life became centered in the camps, a community spirit blossomed. Plantation living had begun to generate a certain sense of pride. A strong work ethic brought more and more high-level schooling, income, and migration to Honolulu and the mainland. The extent of the health care provided is well described by William Dorrance and Francis Morgan in the following overview of a model mid-century plantation complex:

> *"The Hawaiian Commercial and Sugar Company operation in central Maui provided many examples of life at the time. In 1938 this plantation, Hawaii's largest, housed 7,973 employees and dependents in 1,545 company-owned houses in thirty camps distributed over 35,000 acres. Its hospital had a staff of ten, including three physicians. Two power plants supplied electricity to the entire plantation. There were various stores, ten churches, four public schools, three Japanese language schools, and three movie theaters. The largest camps had recreation parks—management was highly organized and efficient, and this also meant, throughout the industry, maintaining the health and welfare of the plantation's large, diverse mixture of inhabitants."* (*Sugar Islands*, p. 131, 2000).

Day care centers, a rarity before WWII in a U. S. territory or on the mainland, allowed working mothers to contribute to plantation productivity as office or field workers. In addition, two nurses and a dietician made regular visits to individual houses in the camps. The provision of plantation medical care was not in any sense quick stop medicine aimed at the indigent. It was the standard care available at the time to the entire community. It was adequately paid for by the appreciable productivity of labor and management.

However, these services were not enough to totally satisfy all workers. Theon Wright, in *The Disenchanted Isles*, tells of the slowly fulminating morass of discontent during these years, fueled by the arrival in 1935 of Jack Hall, a seaman since seventeen, and a skilled labor organizer. The ILWU was then under the control of Harry Bridges who had strong connections with San Francisco's shipping disputes. Despite being accused of Communist ties, Hall and Bridges, organized longshoremen, truck drivers, hotel employees and most importantly, sugar and pineapple field workers into the overwhelming political and financial revolution in Hawaii's history, one that challenged the fifty-year rule of the sugar and pineapple companies known as the "Big Five"—Amfac, Alexander and Baldwin, C. Brewer, Castle and Cooke, and Theo H. Davies. Largely controlled by related owners, these five companies and their management dominated island industry and politics until after WWII. Statehood in 1959 brought new laws to Hawaii that limited interlocking corporate boards and directorships, crippling the power of these giants.

Equally influential in the demise of plantation control of life in the islands was the rapid political rise of highly motivated, competent and well-educated descendants of plantation workers, whose public school and post war GI Bill exposure to the ideas of equality forever changed social and economic relationships in Hawaii as they became judges, legislators and corporate officers.

Earlier, in 1944, the unions had renewed their organizing efforts, focusing on plantation field workers. By 1946, the ILWU had developed great strength throughout the islands. It called a strike for higher pay, better working conditions, fringe benefits, and an end to paternalistic treatment of sugar workers and their families.

As labor and communism were being firmly linked in the media and the public mind, J. C. Carter, the plantation manager at Olokele on Hawaii island wrote:

> *At this time it might be well to say a word in regard to Communism. The subject has been in the headlines of all the national and local papers for sometime...The vicious propaganda drive being put on today does nothing but drive a wedge between the employee and the employer. People*

are told to hate their bosses. They are told that there is no such thing as a good boss. . .We hear talk of sending an army of strikers into the field for a showdown fight against the employers, raising vast sums of money for the "fighting fund." Real honest bargaining between employee and employer will produce far more satisfactory results and good will than all the shouting, spreading hatred and the vicious propaganda we hear today against your bosses. (*Plantation Health,* Annual Report to the Medical Association, 12 Jan. 1948, 12 (I) 36.)

Carter then made a man-to-man plea to his workers. "Let's us look at your bosses here at Olokele. Out of a total of thirty-three supervisors, twenty are island-born men, and some of them right on this plantation. They started at the bottom and through hard work they were promoted to bosses. Let me ask you this—are they no good? The company has no interest in breaking unions. The company wants good relations between your union and your company. We believe you too want good relations between us."

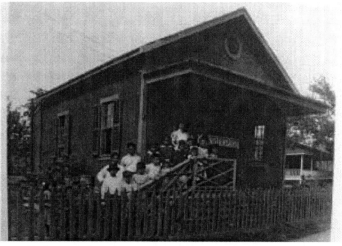

Small, free-standing dispensaries offered outpatient care in convenient locations.

Both sides did, and reason won the day. With negotiations over several years, the pay and benefits of sugar workers continued to increase, and the number of camps, truly landmarks of earlier times, steadily decreased as workers found housing in nearby modern communities.

During this period, Hawaii's plantation workers became the highest paid agricultural workers in the world. By the 1950s, many plantations were breaking up their camps, moving houses to main roads, and selling them and the property to their employees for token amounts, complete with water, phone, electricity and assistance with sewage disposal systems.

These changes all interfaced with generous medical coverage, with hospitalization in community hospitals that gradually changed from plantation ownership and operation to "county hospitals," which later became part of the present state-operated hospital system. Throughout all these changes, both the plantations and the State, to their great credit, maintained private and public medical systems that have to this day assured the great majority of Hawaii's population of at least basic medical care.

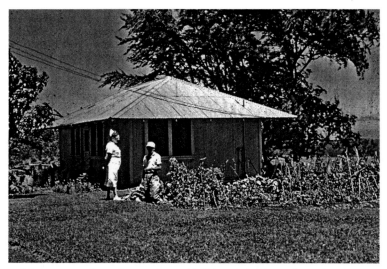

Many nurses from the continental USA married into plantation communities. Plantation- born girls often trained as nurses in Honolulu and returned to work in their local hospitals. Staff was provided with comfortable private housing on plantation hospital grounds at token rates.

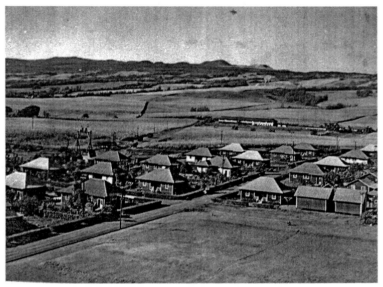

Typical plantation housing after the 1950s.

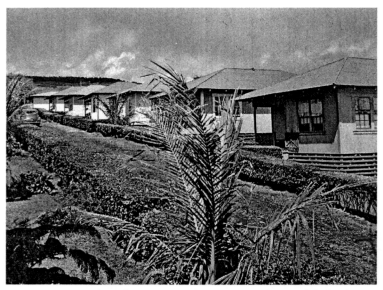

Post WWII employee housing, Hutchinson Sugar Co. Model plumbing, sewage, electrical facilities, clinics, and sports programs graced rural communities.

By WWII, the quality of care provided through the rural medical system in Hawaii far surpassed that available in most mainland states. Beginning in King Kalakaua's reign, parallel with the hiring and maintenance of well-trained physicians by plantation companies, the "Government" or "District" physician was available in most communities, to provide indigent care and Public Health support for government programs. Government physicians were appointed by the Department of Health, or by county governments. Payment was a flat rate per month for which they by contract "attended the indigent, advised on medical matters, and conducted physical examinations as requested by other agencies of the county," as described in a Hawaii County directive.

Plantation and District Physicians together shared patients and problems and were often the same individuals in two roles. The concept of a Public Health Nurse emerged in 1910, leading to the statewide network of Public Health Nursing offices, clinics, and home services that exists to this day. Disease data, immunization records, referrals of problem patients and families, a myriad of well-baby clinics, maternal and child health services originated in these offices, which were run by incredibly dedicated Public Health-trained career nurses.

Monthly clinics were held in plantation dispensaries, school cafeterias, church halls, and gymnasiums, and were arranged in the most distant camps to ensure attendance where patient transport was difficult. Weather was a problem in rainy months, but I recall with wonder the unfailing certainty that despite occasional wind, mud, and pouring rains, the nurse was always there first, with patients registered, lined up, and ready for the doctor.

Paid Public Health nurses were first hired in 1910. Previously, such work was done on a volunteer basis. For several years beginning in 1897, one very public-spirited nurse, Miss Ulrich Thompson served the entire Palama area on Oahu gratis. When the Bureau of Maternal and Child Health was organized in 1926, the nurse services expanded island wide. A Miss Claira Figely was the first supervisor of nurses, followed by Miss Mabel Smyth who was Director of the Bureau of Maternal and Infant Hygiene. Hawaii was the first, and at times the only, state that required formal Public Health training for employment as a Public Health nurse. Although the rural functions of the Public Health nurse have been largely supplanted by direct care in physician's offices, vital community casework is still done by nurses employed by the state Department of Health, an enormous contribution to the public well being.

In a brilliant statement of health care as a fundamental right, the students of Johns Hopkins University School of Hygiene and Public Health noted these elements of a modern, civilized medical system. For most of Hawaii's people today, these aspirations are a reality, the result of social and political amity, sound public health programs, and major industrial support of health insurance.

1992
The International Declaration of Health Rights

We, as people concerned about health improvement in the world, do hereby commit ourselves to advocacy and action to promote the health rights of all human beings. The enjoyment of the highest attainable standard of health is one of the fundamental rights of every human being. It is not a privilege reserved for those with power, money or social standing.

Health is more than the absence of disease, but includes prevention of illness, development of individual potential, and a positive sense of physical, mental and social well-being.

Health care should be based on dialogue and collaboration between citizens, professionals, communities and policy makers. Health services should be affordable, accessible, effective, efficient and convenient.

Health begins with healthy development of the child and a positive family environment. Health must be sustained by the active role of men and women in health and development. The role of women, and their welfare, must be recognized and addressed.

Health care for the elderly should preserve dignity, respect and concern for quality of life and not merely extend life.

Health requires a sustainable environment with balanced human population growth and preservation of cultural diversity.

Health depends on the availability to all people of basic essentials: Food, safe water, housing, education, productive employment, protection from pollution and prevention of social alienation.

Health depends on protection from exploitation without distinction of race, religion, political belief, economic or social condition.

Health requires peaceful and equitable development and collaboration of all peoples.

Created by the students, faculty and alumni on the occasion of the 75th Anniversary of the Johns Hopkins University School of Hygiene and Public Health, April 1992

Suggesting that these landmarks of sound public health policy have largely been met in Hawaii, this statement as part of an article by Dr. John. C. Lewin, Executive Vice President of the California Medical Association was issued in the *American Journal of Surgery*, in February 1994, pg. 227-231.

"In 1974, Hawaii began addressing the problem of health care accessibility. As a result of legislative action, near universal health care coverage has been achieved. These actions include employer mandates to provide adequate health insurance, regulation of insurance products; control of costly health care facilities, and government assistance to those not provided health insurance through employment. By providing primary care, total health care costs are considerably below national average- even though actual cost of living is over 30 percent greater. Public health statistics suggest a healthier population than the national average. This cannot be solely attributed to healthy lifestyle or ethnic mix, but likely involves the effects of the state health care system. Although economically and culturally Hawaii closely resembles the rest of the United States, there has been no evidence of reduced employment due to the 1974 employer healthcare mandate."

CHAPTER 9

Hawaii's Plantation Hospitals

Hawaii's first hospital was a "health station" at Waimea on Hawaii in 1831. The first true hospital was opened in Waikiki only a few years later in 1837 by the U.S. Consul who provided care for ailing seamen, rather than keeping them in a local grog shop which had been their previous abode. Several Oahu hospitals were built during the next decades, some for special purposes such as smallpox and mental disease. In the 1880s, the Hawaiian government extended hospital services to the outer islands to Koloa, Eleele, and Hilo. Koloa had no patients for two years and was closed by the Board of Health in 1903. Various private organizations opened (and subsequently closed) marginal hospitals which were staffed by private or district physicians. Plantation hospitals were started on all the major islands—on Oahu at Ewa, Waialua, Waipahu and Aiea during the 1890s. Before 1900 there were five hospitals on Kauai. Hamakua Mill Company built one at Paauilo in 1902, and at Haiina and Olaa eight years later.

Privately-Operated 'Japanese Hospitals' In Hawaii

An important element in the history of the development of universal medical care in Hawaii that occurred in the early 1900s was the establishment of "Japanese Hospitals." Their advent was artfully described by Dr. Leon H. Bruno in a 1985 publication from Lyman House Memorial Museum, *The Private Japanese Hospital.*

A few excerpts here can only convey a small part of the rich cultural and medical contribution the Japanese physician-owners and operators of these havens of care and support gave to their communities. Dr. Bruno, who was Lyman museum director, wrote:

> "*Accompanying the first shipload of Government contract Japanese immigrant laborers to Hawaii in 1885 on the ship, City of Tokio, was a medical doctor, Dr. Yoshida. The Japanese government, concerned about the health of its citizens traveling to live and work in a foreign and unfamiliar country, insisted on this arrangement. Throughout the history of the Japanese in Hawaii there has been concern about health care. In 1896 a Japanese doctors' association was organized in Hawaii.*
> *Sugar plantations originally provided free health care for their laborers as part of their contracts. The medical personnel, like the fields, the stores, the housing and the recreational facilities, were under the control of the plantation owners. The plantation physicians did not speak Japanese, nor were they Japanese. The type of medical care given was different from what the immigrants knew and had experienced in Japan. It appeared to them to be more impersonal and confusing.*
> *When a Japanese immigrant was hospitalized in a plantation hospital, not only was there a separation from a family if there was one, but there was also a diet different from that to which the Japanese were accustomed. Traditional Japanese customs were seldom considered in plantation or territorial hospitals.*" (*The Private Japanese Hospital*, p. I, 1980).

An interesting solution that would take a little time to blossom, soon surfaced. After the arrival of immigrant labor in Hawaii it soon became clear to many workers and their families that rather than return home, they would face brighter futures by staying on the plantations temporarily, saving, and investing in education or small businesses. Some had firm aspirations to educate their children to become physicians and other leaders. By great sacrifices made by family and friends, plantation-born doctors were trained in Japan and the mainland, returning to their communities to practice. Sensing keenly the cultural gap between their patients and the community hospitals, many established and operated their own hospitals, primarily on Hawaii island. These doctors were highly trained; they and their hospitals were properly licensed.

Although Hilo Hospital and many plantation hospitals were fully operative, and the Japanese doctors had full privileges in them, their patients often chose the small private hospitals because of language problems, dietary preferences, and what they saw as more personalized, sympathetic care. These small, homey hospitals operated from 1907 through 1960, helping to combine ethnic and Western medical practice through the dedication of eleven involved Japanese physicians, five of whom were trained in Japan, and six in the United States.

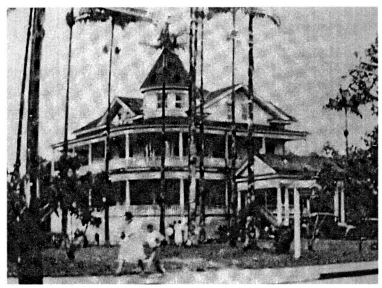

Matsumura Japanese Hospital, Hilo, Hawaii, 1935.
(Old Canario Building).

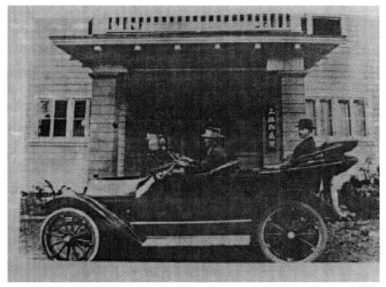

Dr.Chirin Uesu and his driver at the door of Matayoshi Hospital, Hilo, Hawaii, 1914.

Amy J. Hamane, (*Japanese Hospitals of Hilo, 1980*) brings to life details of the typical routine in these small frame structures, which were often modified houses or other buildings.

The doctors were on 24-hour call, seven days a week, and lived within the hospital complex. The members of the family all had responsibilities; several of the wives worked side by side in the operating room and became the physician's most trusted assistant. One wife said that she had had to deliver babies while the doctor was operating on another patient. 'Once they started to come, I couldn't tell them to wait!' Other staff, especially young nurses, lived at the hospital and were on 24-hour call. There was usually a handyman who was responsible for grounds and buildings plus general errand running, often accompanying the doctor on house calls. (Hamane, Japanese Hospitals of Hilo, quoted in The Private Japanese Hospital, July, 1985).

Everyday practices in these small, homelike hospitals were unique in Hawaii, comparable in many ways with present activities found in the hospitals of remote Western Pacific islands. For example, patients often paid for services in food—fruits, or fish or with work instead of cash. Hospital gardens and chicken coops were common. The menu was Asian, becoming more Western in later times. Family members shared patients' rooms, helping with patient care, a concept being quietly revived as sophisticated urban hospitals today face crippling nursing shortages.

Patients were cared for regardless of means. The doctors worked quite independently of each other, even though "groups" of Western physicians were forming around them. The Japanese doctors were greatly respected in the community for many reasons beyond medicine, as community leaders, sage advisers, and gracious examples of humanitarian values.

One of the most memorable of these gentlemen was one with whom fate decreed that I "cross swords" in the late 1950s over the issue of fluoridation in the prevention of dental decay. My fervent but truly gentlemanly clinical opponent was Dr. Toshio Kutsanai, a highly regarded Hilo, Hawaii, physician who was born in 1901 in Niulii, a part of Kohala. Through great family support he was educated in Honolulu, attended Northwestern University, and trained in Cook County Hospital in Chicago. When he was thirty-two years old he returned to Kohala to visit his mother's grave. Recognition of his clinical acumen at our Kohala hospital led to his setting up an office in a rented cottage and soon moving to nearby Honokaa where he bought and operated a precariously situated hillside hospital with an outside stairway. According to an account Dr. Bruno included in *The Private Japanese Hospital*, his staff consisted of a laundry woman, two cooks, a yardman, and a former machinist who took x-rays, worked in the laboratory, assisted in surgery, and was Dr. Kutsanai's driver.

Dr. Kutsanai's final practice years were in Hilo where I tangled with him in the media and in friendly arguments over the preventive use of fluoride tablets for our plantation children in a program we launched in the 1950s to prevent tooth decay. At Kohala Sugar Company's expense, and with the help of the Dental Division of the Department of Health, we had set up a treatment and control group to measure the effects of fluoride tablets. All was going well until Dr. Kutsanai's popularity among the Kohala population and his public blasts of "rat poison" blew our well planned program out of the water. A few parents, however, persisted in giving their children the daily tablets. One family came to our dispensary long afterward with two siblings, an older one whose unfluoridated teeth had formed before we started our tablet-ingestion program, and a younger one who had been given the tablets—to show us the marked difference—the treated one, had no decay- and the untreated one had several badly rotted teeth. Unfortunately, our few subjects were not enough to let us publish firm statistical conclusions.

The fluoride battle persists today despite sound evidence supporting the safety and effectiveness of fluoride ingestion in the prevention of dental decay. Although Dr. Kutsanai, the media, the Department of Health, and I had many a fine fuss over all this, I remember the doctor as a kindly capable person with the interests of his many loyal followers firmly at heart.

Plantation Hospitals

For some sixty years beginning in the 1890s plantation

hospitals and their dispensaries were the heart of rural care in Hawaii. Originally, the hospitals were single-story frame buildings with spacious rooms housing surgical and obstetrical areas that opened onto wide, screened lanais. In later years modest laboratory and x-ray facilities, diathermy and EKG equipment were added.

Facilities in smaller hospitals were not necessarily "state of the art" but met most community hospital needs. Outpatient care was provided in a "dispensary" in, or very near, the hospital. After plantation ownership and operation began to be replaced by county or state support, and after the Hill-Burton legislation of 1946 provided matching Federal grants for hospital construction, these picturesque older centers with their open areas, gardens, covered walkways, and latticed ventilation panels, faded from the architectural scene, replaced by winter-proof building styles from mainland states. The new structures were serviceable and fire resistant, but lacked the unique charm of single-wall board and batten "plantation carpentry" so typical of the earlier buildings.

The ancient rambling frame structure that was the Kohala Hospital I first knew in 1956 was of an ideal design for both patients and staff—a "T" in shape, with service areas, kitchen, staff dining room, laboratory and x-ray in the standing part, the patient rooms and wards across the top of the "T, " with the nursing station near the crossing point. Inpatient rooms, surgery, and the delivery room were only a few steps steps from the nurses' station.

The staff dining room was small, with plantation-style horizontally sliding windows and lace curtains, an ancient oak Victorian dining table and chairs, and a classic serving buffet with a mirror and proper doilies under the silver plated coffee service prominently displayed on top. The setting was much

much more that of a friendly home than a sterile hospital milieu.

The foundations of these buildings were typically post and block. In the four or five foot clearance space between the building floor and the bare ground were decades of stored junk—old bed frames, gas cans, pipe, lumber, paint, roofing iron, gurney parts, hopelessly broken wheelchairs, and other nameless relics of the past. This intriguing jungle of memories was also home to assorted cats who were, when not pampered by our cook, our major rodent control corps. The space beneath the building was an underworld, artistically hidden behind an openwork frame created by a carpenter's choice of one-inch lathe strips—horizontal or crisscross—a sure feature of classic plantation carpentry still found under wooden camp housing, utility buildings and sheds in the islands. Include the single-walled construction, rusting corrugated iron roof, outside plumbing and wiring, and brightly contrasting colors for walls and window frames, and we have the classic plantation architectural scene. Over time, governance of the hospitals varied from outright ownership and operation by the plantations through a period of takeover by the County in which they were located, and finally, in recent years, by the State of Hawaii. By 1943, multiple small 20-to 40-bed plantation hospitals near larger community centers were starting to merge into multi-specialty centers with "open staffing," welcoming all community physicians. Smaller hospitals became long-term care centers with a limited emergency room, and most remain so today, requiring increasingly costly emergency transport services, usually by helicopter.

CHAPTER 10

Universal Health Care, Plantation Style

In 1935, social workers and teachers in the islands proposed medical insurance that in 1938 became one of the first plans in the nation to offer comprehensive coverage for physician services, home and office visits for minor problems, and hospitalization for major illness and surgery. This was the birth of the Hawaii Medical Service Association (HMSA), which later became a major player in both private and plantation-funded medical care. With the waning of most plantation-based industry in Hawaii, many plantation workers became members of HMSA plans, either through new employers' contracts or as individual families, with small co-pay contributions—charged mostly to discourage over-utilization.

Although the growth and success of major clinics and hospitals on larger islands has attracted highly competent specialty physicians, special nursing staff, technicians and professional administrators, gaps have developed in the universal coverage that graced the plantation medical systems in earlier times. Public Health Nurses and community health centers take up some of the "slack" for the indigent, and extensive State programs continue to bring care to the economic fringe of Hawaii society.

Far different from complex clinics in larger centers, Kohala Dispensary, during my residence in the 1950s was a typical model of rural outpatient care. It stood only a few yards away from the County-operated hospital and it was owned and run by the Kohala Sugar Company, a subsidiary of Castle and Cooke, the parent company. Management never in any way interfered with patient care or expenditures—adequate resources were ours on request. The County government was equally bountiful with hospital funding and staffing; the local Public Health Nurse shared our office and supplies, and no rent or bookkeeping cluttered our relationships.

In the post-war years, there were usually two physicians employed by the plantation. Dr. Barton Eveleth and I shared the Kohala area practice for seventeen years from 1956 to 1973.

Island plantation physicians over the years numbered in the hundreds—often moving from one plantation to another, some serving several at once, particularly in later years when agricultural company mergers became common. Many doctors served short terms, moving to Honolulu or the mainland. Others chose fifteen to thirty year stays in a remarkably stable employment milieu. Common to most, as gauged by their life stories is the aura of dedication that colored all their activities, particularly in the early years of crippling isolation.

Dr. James Wight and "Greenbanks"

Mirroring the happy fate of my chance encounter that led to Kohala plantation life, the destiny of Dr. James Wight, Kohala's first physician, hung on the slimmest thread of maritime fortune.

Leaving his practice in Australia in 1850 to seek his future in the California gold fields, his plans suddenly were changed when he was shipwrecked with his family at Mahukona, a tiny bay on the north tip of Hawaii island. Dr. Wight and his very pregnant wife made it ashore with a young child that died in her arms. He and his family lost everything except several cases of onions that reached shore with them and some salvaged timbers. A doctor was badly needed in nearby Kohala. Selling the onions at a good price, he found housing, and set up practice in the back of a small store. Early success led to opening a drug store, then developing sugar and cattle interests on his 3,282 acres of land which he soon acquired by skillful practice, thrift, and productive investment. At one point in his career he owned 17,000 acres on various islands.

The Wight family lived for many years in high style in an ornate Victorian home built about 1870 on a 22-acre estate known as Greenbank ("Greenbanks" to the local population). Despite galling travel conditions guests from all over Hawaii were entertained. The doctor finally became a member of the House of Nobles, dying in 1905 at the age of 91. The Wights had thirteen children, six of whom died in childhood.

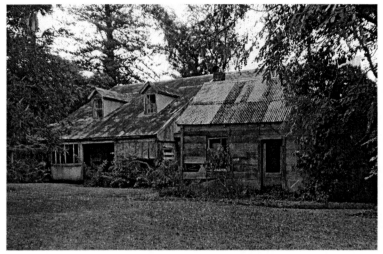

Greenbank, plantation physician, Dr. James Wight's Kohala, Hawaii, residence. Abandoned, fully furnished, after 1905, the mansion finally succumbed to termites and vandals in the early 1970s. Ladies would arrive in early years from all over the island by carriage or horseback for parties, dressed in formal Victorian dress and hip boots, against dust and ankle deep mud.

In 1882, during the formative years of his household, a natural stone figure with a malevolent face was found near the cliffs at Pololu Valley, a deep Kohala gorge. The figure was brought by the local people to Mrs. Wight who set it up in her yard at Greenbank. Immediate, serious family turmoil began. There was illness, insanity, and deep family hatred, and the banishment of one son. The family never recovered amity, and in anger went its several ways.

In 1927, a Wight granddaughter, Amy Rice, thinking to end the strife, quietly arranged to have the figure transported to the Bishop Museum in Honolulu where it sits snarling today in the courtyard. Soon afterward, the family abandoned the entire estate, leaving only a little money to maintain the yard.

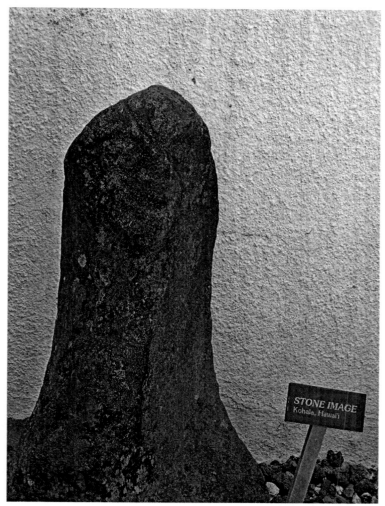

Stone figure from Greenbank estate, Kohala, Hawaii. (In Bernice Bishop Museum courtyard, Honolulu, Hawaii.)

By the 1950s, the fully furnished, beautifully appointed home had become a termite-eaten derelict, with broken windows, falling plaster, smashed furniture, invading creepers, an upside-down piano, and collapsing floors.

In 1973, the estate was was sold in a family auction to Mr. and Mrs Wilford Hunt who were family members, and again in 1983 to John Dowie, a real estate broker from Spain. Beyond the tragic aura of the crumbling mansion and the feuding family, 1990 marked the final curse of the stone figure, when the U.S. Customs Service seized the property, claiming it was finally purchased with drug money. It now belongs to the State of Hawaii, Department of Land and Natural Resources, and is listed as a historic site. Historic indeed.

The buildings have been demolished; only rare hundred-year-old plantings and the tiny family cemetery remain.

After Dr. Wight, other physicians came to the district, and after 1862, each cared for the workers of a string of small independent Kohala plantations which finally combined in 1937 to form the Kohala Sugar Company, under the parent company, Castle and Cooke. There was one hospital, and the dispensary that was built just before WWII just in time for fate to drop a heavy surprise on another Kohala- bound doctor.

Dr. Ivar Larsen, from Cornell, was getting some clinical experience in Hilo, Hawaii, as part of his post-graduate training on December 7, 1941. He was caught under martial law and sent to Kohala where he was the only physician through 1946, with no backup except one registered nurse, and the chief nurse at the hospital who had married the plantation manager.

Dr. Larsen recalled having to perform surgeries at Kohala Hospital with only his nurse assistant. He was provided with a telephone at home for emergencies. He delivered some of his own children, and his wife did not leave the island for three years. In 1945, when 200 Filipinos came to Kohala, he did physical exams on all of them. One in ten had syphilis. The treatment was bismuth since penicillin was not yet available, although Dr. Larsen's brother, Dr. Nils Larsen, who was in Honolulu, sent him cultures from which he grew the mold and soaked gauze in the culture medium to use on open wounds. Occasional transfusions were done, direct from patient to patient, with rubber tubing, two needles, and a rubber bulb squeeze pump. Leaving Kohala after the war for orthopedic training, Dr. Larsen spent many more years in a Honolulu practice. His Kohala patients loved him and often spoke of his years in the district.

One night when I was still very new in Kohala, I was called to the hospital to see a Filipino man of about fifty in a coma who had been brought in by his housemates who said he had been that way all day. When I walked into the room, the diagnosis may as well have been written on the wall—the room reeked of acetone and the man looked as if he might be breathing his last. They had already tested his urine, which was "loaded" with sugar. Clearly he was in a severe diabetic coma. I asked for bicarbonate solution to give by vein to combat this obvious acidosis, but there was none available. We grubbed around in the laboratory cupboards and found a large glass funnel that we could hook up to some old, buff-colored laboratory tubing that we could slip over the hub of a needle. We filled the funnel with tap water (at least, it had been boiled) and with nothing else sterilized, ran the water into an arm vein while I stirred in Arm and Hammer bicarbonate of soda directly out of the box with a tongue blade for a scoop. Dose??? I never knew, but it must have been enough. With slugs of insulin, and a lot more bicarbonate, he lived to resume work and chicken fighting weekends.

"Vun Month Nearer the Grave"

Kohala dispensary, owned by the Kohala Sugar Company, a Castle and Cooke subsidiary, was a classic plantation-built, one-story frame building about the size of a very small house, on the single- lane access road to the hospital. Four or five steps led to a narrow open lanai across the front, with small wooden benches and a "two by four" wood railing. Patients, mostly plantation workers or their families, arrived by plantation truck that collected them from the camps.

Occupying the benches outside on the lanai, or inside in a square room holding twenty to thirty people of all ages, conditions, and origin, patients awaited their turns to be seen. Contrasts in dress and wealth were fascinating. Our practice in later years even included the sophisticated guests of Rockefeller's Mauna Kea Beach Hotel—ponchos and muddy boots of our field workers made a fetching background for Gucci bags, miniskirts, and designer shoes.

Periodically, when one of us was on vacation, Dr. Sergei Ross, an elderly Russian physician who, with his wife, had escaped the Russian revolution by hiking over the Himalayas with the government in hot pursuit, would "cover" for us. His unfailing humor was only matched by his large paunch accented by a white coat, his deep bass voice, erudition, and exotic accent. In the midst, one day, of our watchful waiting-room audience, he strode out of his office, and noting the month on the wall calendar needed changing, ripped it off the wall with a dramatic sweep, and the memorable words, "VUN MONTH NEARER THE GRAVE!" He was a true character who must have outlived most of his Soviet tormentors.

Time seemed suspended in our lush green world between the Kohala Mountains and the sea as weeks, months and years passed. Our work schedule was stable and reasonably regular—one half day off midweek, then covering the weekend for hospital and dispensary day and night—really 84-hour weeks but with much of our time spent just waiting for something to happen that could lie anywhere between happy challenge and tragedy.

Patients had no appointments. At the dispensary a midday break was routine and welcome, often with lunch and siesta. Some days a hundred patients would be seen, using several examining rooms and four faithful, resourceful, local plantation workers' wives as aides paid by the plantation management. Clinical life was good. Our relationships with patients were cemented by our knowing practically all the patients and their ailments, and by their trust in the medical system and us. We were free to refer very serious cases when necessary, and occasionally, sent them to Hilo by car, or to Honolulu by air. DC3 service into Upolu Point was sometimes available with teeth-chattering landings on the short bumpy airstrip, and the Coast Guard would occasionally land a C130 for us on request for a Honolulu transfer.

A Nearly Idyllic Life Style

One dismal wet afternoon when I was working alone at the dispensary, after having served about sixty patients that day, I was suddenly called over to the hospital. All the dispensary patients had been seen except one, which the nurse had put up in stirrups in the back room to await a pelvic examination. My hospital call was urgent and rather long—when it was finished, I collapsed into my jeep and went straight home. At dinner the phone rang. A voice on the other end said, "Hey doc, this is Maizie. Did you forget me this afternoon?" My reply was a choked, "Oh." Then, "Oh God Maize, I forgot you were waiting." Patients were kinder in those days. Maize said, "Doc, don't worry. When your girls left, I waited for a long time, then figured you wouldn't be back, climbed down out of the stirrups, dressed, and went around and closed the windows, turned out the lights, locked the door, and went home." Truly, as doctors, we weren't perfect, but we surely enjoyed our world of forgiving patients.

Our medical record keeping at Kohala was primitive but worked. We would write brief notes on a small sheet which also ordered medications from what we termed the "pharmacy window"—a square hole through a wall into the "drug room," presided over by a bright young girl whose pharmacy training was from visiting drug salesmen, the Physicians' Desk Reference (it was thinner then), the Merck Manual, and what it said on the bottle. A typist typed our clinical notes onto three by five cards, which fit quite nicely into several shoeboxes. "Modern" office conveniences were an old Remington typewriter, a hand-cranked pencil sharpener, a large clanking adding machine, and the phone, which usually worked. Patient confidentiality problems and HIPPA (current mind-bending Federal rules for medical record keeping) lay a half-century away.

All care for plantation workers and their families was provided under the plantation salary paid to us by Kohala Sugar Company. Non-plantation patients paid directly or through HMSA in later years. The medications we dispensed were provided free to plantation employees. What we collected from private patients was part of the physicians' perquisites, which included a four-wheel drive vehicle with full maintenance, malpractice insurance, and for each of us, a comfortable home for $65 a month, gardener, maid, one-month vacation a year, and three months every third year, plus transportation costs to the mainland for continuing medical education.

Plantation physicians' salaries were modest, but living was very reasonable and relatively simple. Our entertainment was our romantic, complex environment, the starry night sky, memorable forages into the gulches and mountains, a sturdy boat and the ever-present sea with its mysteries. We had good friends, music, and half dozen exotic cultures to explore, time for reading and research, and a "laid-back" lifestyle that often offered a touch of unexpected humor.

When my two boys were at just the right age for such things, I bought a surplus WWII weapons carrier rigged as a crane, with winch, and heavy lifting tackle—perfect men's toys, which we kept in our carport. About three o'clock one morning, the police called me to say there had been a bad car accident a few miles away, and would I come out right away. I asked if I should stop at the hospital to pick up splints or anything we might need. After a long silence, the answer on the phone was a rather tentative, "well, no, doc, nobody was hurt, but the car is upside down and the road is blocked and we wondered if you'd bring your crane!" My kids and I went right out and moved the wreck; in one of those rare family adventures money cannot buy.

Laughs came easily in our close-to nature environment. What I remember as a wry lesson in bovine nutrition involved a certain cow.

Cows are calm, thoughtful creatures, seldom bent on mischief—or so I thought, based on boyhood Ohio farm experience. One cow was an exception. One day, I drove out to a tiny tofu factory that was located in an old house on a country road, to learn about tofu. An elderly Japanese lady kindly showed me around and explained how she made it.

When I went in to her little factory, I had parked my shiny Buick convertible beside the road near a presumably contented cow tethered to a stake driven into the shallow grassy roadside ditch. After an hour or so, I came back to the car, only to find the entire cloth top was missing. A large piece of it was hanging out of Bossy's mouth as she chomped down the last piece of evidence, which had been nicely soaked the day before with linseed oil top-dressing. The tasty waterproofing must have triggered her gourmet interest.

When I reporting her bovine "dining experience" to the insurance agent in Hilo, he thought I was crazy. It took three months and an agent in New York City who probably had never seen a cow, to pay the claim. County life has its risks.

Kohala Hospital, Suspended in Time

For our 17 years of Kohala practice, Kohala Hospital rounds began precisely at 0800 when Dr. Barton Eveleth, my partner, had finished his second cup of coffee, which ended, for the staff doctors (all two of us) and the nurses, our daily morning meeting that took place in the tiny hospital dining room. Once in the sixties, the first of the Joint Commission of Accreditation of Healthcare Organizations types appeared with briefcase and forms on our bucolic hospital scene, and upon their inquiring about how often the hospital had staff meetings, and what the physician attendance record was, we were all amused to respond by pegging it at 100 percent about twenty days a month, probably a national record.

Morning conversational fare over coffee included plantation scuttlebutt, politics, a joke or two, and patient issues, with occasional special treats from the kitchen, all presided over by our starched, immaculately uniformed and coifed combination hospital superintendent, anesthetist, chief nurse, and fiscal officer who deigned to be known as "Flossie." This delightful customary start of each day was ruffled at one point by my temporary mainland haole effort at "continuous improvement" with the introduction of our listening to an audiotape, which might drone on about the clinical uses of a mass spectrometer while we were just trying to get our centrifuge to run.

After coffee, in a proper procession, led by our lady Hospital Superintendent, we would stop at the desk for the chart buggy that had one slightly flat wheel, and with the formality of rounds at the Massachusetts General Hospital, visit each room and bed, greeting our patients with *"zao chen hao, ohio gozaimasu, aloha kakahiaka,"* or whatever morning greeting seemed most gracious.

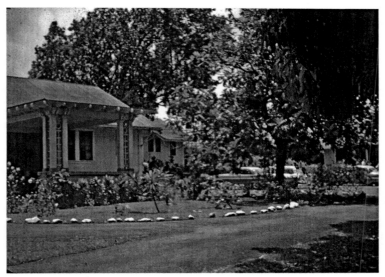

Kohala Hospital, Kapaau, Hawaii, 1956. Replaced by stone and steel facility in 1962. Operation, as with most plantation hospitals was taken over by the county or state government.

Patients were clean, shaven, polite, and seemed always to be in good cheer. Discourse was, of course, in pidgin, the indispensable Pacific Islands' creole, with assists from our multiethnic staff. One unusual 92-year-old black gentleman known as "Daddy," who spoke the King's English, even regaled us daily about his having been a coachman for King Kalakaua.

One form of preventive medicine we often practiced was

to hospitalize older Filipino men for a day or two just to give them a few good meals and a nice nurse to talk to, a practice that would buoy them up for months.

Some of the laboratory aspects of our practice were a challenge. Many of our Filipino workers enjoyed raw meat dishes, or were recent arrivals from rural areas in the Western Pacific. These individuals often had an impressive burden of intestinal parasites. Pork and beef tapeworms were legion, as were Ascaris, fine, fat, foot-long roundworms. Patients would come in to say they had passed something suspicious, usually described as "da kine eggs." This usually triggered some medicine from our nurse, and a large empty jar with the patient's name on it. In a day or so, our usual reward was the jar full of tapeworm, which necessitated our curious but rather brief attention to several feet of the creature to find the very narrow head where the hooks are. The search is essential to a cure, for if the head is missing, all is for naught, and the worm regrows and lives on in its mobile home. The critical lack in our early laboratory of a fume hood, a small, enclosed work area with a fan and a stack for ventilation, rather dimmed our enthusiasm for the technical demands of laboratory parasitology.

A Precarious Balance

For many quietly productive decades stable, smoothly running plantation medical systems such as ours were not ruinously expensive for the plantation companies. Total expenditures in the early and middle years was tolerable, as modern very high cost interventions and medications had not yet surfaced. Later, as hospital costs rose, the shifts to outside insurance, such as the popular HMSA plans, were briefly able to prolong most plantation coverage.

However, the original "cradle-to-grave" medical system,

excellent as it was, was fated to collapse along with many other relatively positive elements of recent plantation life that have for most areas, been replaced by urban development, conflicting values, lost jobs and security, and in many areas, a scattered population. The fragmentation of what was once broad healthcare coverage now includes even the serious lack of specialist care in larger centers. Truly, "the old order changeth."

CHAPTER 11

Plantation Life Inspires An Alternative Medicine Study

Another unexpected thread of fate that greatly influenced my Hawaii clinical life, wound subtly among the patients I saw daily. In our small, informally run hospital, beside delicious homemade snacks in the bedside stands, very often there was a little bottle of homemade medicine, something to rub on, some leaves in a bag, or a lomi lomi stick for self-massage; all these, of course, were part of the rather quietly active cultural medicinal practices of our very mixed ethnic groups. Every day too, the dispensary practice revealed cherished alternative medications and beliefs that were far from our standard care.

In addition to the specific cultural practices of the Hawaiians, Filipinos, and Portuguese, the area's Japanese Sensei or Buddhist priests were often knowledgeable in local herbal materials. The Hawaiian families had trusted healers whose skills they prized, such as Thomas Soloman, Kohala Hospital's ambulance driver, and Heloke Mookini, a very wise gentleman in his eighties, who was the Kahuna Nui, or guardian priest of Mookini Heiau, a 1500 year old stone religious structure in the district, once used for sacrifices, prayers, and healing. Friendships with these knowledgeable people soon led to long conversations, inquiries, and collections of plant and sea materials for later analysis.

In understanding the medical characteristics of the community, Dr. Eveleth and I felt it essential to explore, to the extent possible to us, the alternative medicine practices in use at the time. The evaluation of alternative medical practices is an unfinished task to this day. What has been studied to date, whether found to be useful or not, merits disclosure. The saga of our Kohala research activities is presented here with that intent, and with the belief that discussion of a health-care system should ideally report the activity and results of any associated research program.

My first useful employment in my training years was as an assistant to a pharmacologist working in a dingy basement, studying the effects on rats and cats of stilbesterol, an artificial female hormone made in the laboratory. This early background was not exactly Nobel-level work, but it provided the grounding for long lasting research interests.

In the early 1960s, my physician partner at Kohala and I were well aware of the record of excellent clinical research done at Ewa Plantation many years before, and Dr. Eveleth had already begun a systematic recording of some of the reported uses of plant medicines among our patients. Interest in ethnopharmaceutic discovery was burgeoning worldwide, and the National Cancer Institute was funding large-scale surveys of natural products in the search for anticancer compounds. With our daily interaction with actual local ethnic practices, it seemed an excellent opportunity to study to the best of our ability the plant materials available to us.

In 1962, Dr. Bart Eveleth and I, after several months of training in the methods of drug extraction and animal testing with Dr. James Dille at the University of Washington School of Medicine, set up a small data bank and laboratory at Kohala Hospital.

In 1965, the invaluable support of my receiving a faculty appointment to the Department of Pharmacology, chaired by Dr. Bert Lum, at the University of Hawaii, financing from Kahua Ranch in North Kohala, The American Cancer Society, and a Federal Grant to the University School of Medicine, made it possible for us to gather, grind, extract and screen by animal tests and cultures, for possible medicinal activity many of the materials we found in common use by our Kohala patients, and others in various Pacific islands.

After basic extraction and mouse tests in Kohala, chemically interesting extracts were sent for further study to the University of Hawaii in Honolulu, where a large Public Health Service grant-funded study of natural products from the Pacific Basin was under way. In this program, over 1000 species of medicinal plants, fungal cultures, marine algae, marine bacteria and marine invertebrates were collected, identified, studied, extracted and tested for pharmacologic activity which included antiviral, antitumor, antimicrobial, antifungal, antifertility, and general nervous system effects on animals and appropriate organisms.

During the years this program was operative, it was my good fortune (threads of fate again) to spend several months in Tahiti and on the Great Barrier Reef in Australia collecting information and specimens for the study. Ultimately, several of our marine specimens showed remarkable antitumor activity on some animal tumors but fell short of National Cancer Institute criteria for clinical use. A summary review of the entire project and a listing of the materials assayed is in Appendix I of this book.

Research occasionally requires some borderline chicanery. In our new hospital, built in 1962, formula for bottle-fed babies in the nursery was being prepared as needed in a pristine baby-formula preparation room. We coveted the room, which was complete with sinks, super lighting, refrigerators, and furnishings to use as a laboratory. After a short period of wallowing in envy, a solution came to mind. Freeing the room by simply ordering prepared ready-to-use baby formula, we commandeered, presto, our prize workplace. It was cheaper for the hospital not to wash bottles, the babies were happy, the Similac baby formula company was happy, and we were in business, setting up our equipment. My first acquisition was a donated desk.

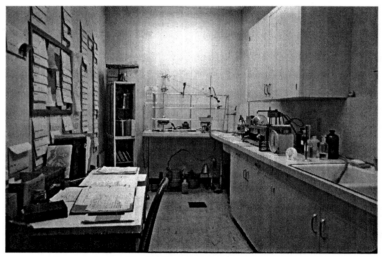

"Baby-formula room," Kohala Hospital, converted to natural products laboratory, 1960.

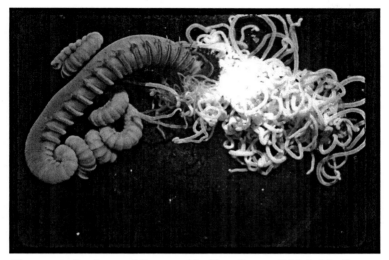

Clam worm, Lanice conchilega, used by Hawaiians on Molokai for "cancer treatment." White tentacles were cooked in an iron skillet and fed to the patient. Tests revealed no anti-cancer activity in the worm itself, but there was a significant effect on a mouse tumor, apparently from algae in the worm that it had consumed as food.

To prepare our plant, animal, or insect materials for testing, we usually ground them in an ordinary Sears Roebuck blender in water or ethyl alcohol, or ligroine, a substance rather like gasoline, used to extract fats. This mush-like material was then filtered and concentrated in some very fancy glassware on a lab stand called a "monkey rack" Then we used a rotating evaporator to produce a little bottle of extract that could be injected into or fed to a mouse or rat, or used for other purposes. The alarming odors we could produce in the building were frequently a source of considerable hospital staff interest.

Despite our sparkling glassware, orderly chemical bottles, and humming equipment, we were still in rural Kohala, not a big-city medical center, so minor fiascos sometimes occurred.

One night, the thirty white mice in our mouse colony arranged among themselves to escape from their cage, creating a brief furor by invading the patients' rooms, climbing the drapes, and running back and forth along the curtain rods. Some vanished into the cane fields outside to breed with wild mice, whose progeny, if they have a mouse theology, will no doubt celebrate the miracle of their escape. Our patients in their rooms, good country dwellers, saw the humor of that night, probably thinking, "that crazy haole doctor." Elsewhere today, we would probably be sued for "emotional distress."

During several years of collection of information and specimens of medicinal plants, curious and cooperative patients in our practice wanted to show us for themselves that certain medicinal plants they knew about "would work." I recall one impressive example of an effective home remedy when a miserably itching case of resolving chickenpox was much comforted by a "washing down" with a diluted brew of Popolo berries (Solanum nigrum) which probably worked as a mild astringent.

Another day someone suggested we go out to one of the gulches where an old gentleman lived who reportedly made a potent "tonic" which he regularly distributed to his friends. On arrival, we were ushered into an old shed containing a small barrel with a removable wooden lid that contained the magic concoction. Our friend, of widely mixed ethnic background, enthusiastically scooped out a large dipperful of the dark green liquid in the barrel which we drank while he described the recipe—several hats full of various leaves, water, whiskey, and the final critical ingredient. Describing that, he said, "In China, we put in tiger head, here no more tiger, so I put in pussy-cat."

Although nearly everyone—all the various ethnic population groups—swore by guava shoot tea for diarrhea, we never could relate severity of stools to dosage or a half dozen other variables, to pin down whether guava is really effective. Most common diarrheas are self-limiting.

On one occasion, we had a gentleman in the hospital for an injury who was a more or less controlled diabetic about fifty years old—controlled with a modest daily dose of long-acting insulin. His daughter wanted us to try to manage his glucose levels instead with a "tea" she prepared from a greyish-green, low-lying plant related to the sages. The Hawaiians usually call the plant Ahinahina, or botanically speaking, *Artemesia australis*, a common endemic Hawaiian species. We agreed to try it.

On hospital admission with no treatment, our patient's blood sugars ran about 260 and his pulse around 70. After a brief observation, we started him on his daughter's homemade extract, 120 cc (1/2 cup) twice a day. Although his blood sugar remained at about the same level for the 15 days of treatment, while taking her tea, his pulse rate fell from around 70 at rest to 50 to 60. Otherwise, no electrocardiographic or other effects on his heart were noted. Put back on insulin, his sugar fell to its usual treatment levels of around 120. We found later that Orinase, an antidiabetic prescription taken by mouth, did not affect his blood sugar either.

Curiosity, it is said, killed the cat. My good friend and colleague, Dr. Bart Eveleth, and I decided to try some of the big jug of the leftover extract that was still in the hospital refrigerator. After a few days of daily blood sugar determinations to set a "base line," we both started on the same dose as our patient and had the lab tech continue to do blood sugars on us. They stayed unchanged; but after some days, we both noted some confusion, weakness, and loss of libido. We dumped the rest down the sink. Our notes however, suggested that because of the apparent heart-rate effect on our patient, and the plant's known content of a neurotoxin, it may be worthy of further study.

Shift Of Our Study to Marine Animals

Our most interesting and chemically rewarding materials were not the many plant specimens assayed but the sea creatures we included. A Hawaiian fisherman told us of the Kumimi crab, thought by our informants to be *Petrolisthes coccineus*, described in early Hawaiian writings as violently poisonous, but which after appropriate extraction, proved to be entirely innocuous to mice. As with many crabs worldwide, toxicity of the tissues of the crab turned out to be limited to certain seasons and the crab's periodic ingestion of toxic algae in its feeding habits.

The search for medicinally useful natural products is often made more difficult because of the many different common names a plant or sea animal may have, or complexities in its actual scientific classification. We often found two or three names in use for what we thought was the same plant.

Additionally, a plant may vary widely in its chemical content with season, differing soil conditions, and other variables that occur during its collection and storage.

Well into our study, Dr. Eveleth and I and the researchers at the Pharmacology Department at the School of Medicine in Honolulu were struck by the finding that most of the soft corals, jellyfish and clam worms we studied had clear-cut biologic effects on our animals, usually anti-tumor activity in mice. Except for Kava, a social drink with sedative properties used throughout the Pacific, and imported species such as the castor plant and Oleander, it was rare to find significant activity in Hawaiian plants. In this three-year University of Hawaii study, it is remarkable that the "classical pharmacologic assay" testing the effects of extracts from 1,089 plant, fungus, and animal sources, showed only 5 percent of them with activity of any sort, except temporary blood pressure reduction. This suggests the rarity of very active medicinal substances in the Polynesian pharmacopoeia, despite wide ethno-pharmacologic interest, and the popularity of the region's many plant materials in alternative medical treatment.

Two notable exceptions however, are *limu make o Hana*, well known in Hawaiian tradition as a deadly poison found in *Palythoa toxica*, a sea anemone, and a plant used for stunning fish in tide pools. This plant, *Tephrosia piscatorium*, or *Auhuhu*, contains tephrosin, a close chemical relative of rotenone, familiar to us in insect spray. Each of these materials has been studied extensively, and there may be possible medical uses for compounds in the anemone.

Published lists of Polynesian plants used by healers, and their purported value, grace the literature, but the difficulty of identifying with reasonable certainty the plants used, and of equal importance, what the disorders treated actually were, makes most such publications very difficult to assess clinically.

External applications, such as of *noni* fruit or leaves, *laukahi*, *kowali*, or other pounded material were common among the earliest recorded treatments, as were emetics and cathartics. External applications may well have had local effects and the results of emetics or cathartics were obvious. Semantic nonsense such as "cleansing the blood" as commonly claimed for some alternative treatments is meaningless physiologically.

With no knowledge in precontact cultures of organ or tissue pathology, and their lists of treatment indications often directed only at a broad range of symptoms of undetermined origin, it is probable that then, as now, only random or very little pharmacologic activity actually occurred when remedies prepared from plants and sea materials were used.. Most benefits, if any, were very likely psychosomatic, effectively reinforced by the Kahuna's revered status and interpersonal skills.

The paucity of toxicity in the indigenous Polynesian plants assayed supports this view as most pharmacologically active materials show toxicity at large doses, whereas only a handful of plants of island origin have, so for, shown any remarkable effects in laboratory assays. This general lack of poisonous substances in indigenous plants may have an interesting evolutionary history.

Most pharmacologically active materials such as digitalis and quinine are poisons if ingested in large doses, but may be medically useful in small amounts. Plants lacking poisons in their parts are rarely effective as medicines, but may serve well as foods. That almost no indigenous plants contain toxic compounds explains why they have little or no physiological or medicinal effects.

Because of Hawaii's geographic isolation, there have been, over the eons, relatively few environmental threats to Hawaiian plants from insect or animal attack. They have not had to develop potent alkaloids, phenols, resins, or other chemical defenses that are common in the plant life of the teeming jungles of the large tropical continents. And so it is not surprising that detailed testing reveals that our benign endemic flora has little or no toxicity, and thus shows little potential medicinal activity in classical pharmacologic screening studies.

Despite these considerations, Kava (Piper methysticum), and Aloe (not indigenous) are still studied, primarily because of their wide social and commercial uses. Noni, because of past reports of possible antitumor properties, is the focus of a cancer study at the Cancer Center of Hawaii. The algae, of which there are some extremely toxic local species, are too of considerable interest.

In the years since we concluded our studies, drug research has become vastly more productive through proteomics, genomics, and incredibly powerful microchip assays. All these have vastly outdistanced classical pharmacologic methods of drug discovery. As with thousands of other potential sources of possibly useful natural products, the materials covered in the University of Hawaii's 1960s study should be reviewed and rescreened with modern technology, particularly the marine components, with extension to the hundreds of yet unassayed forms.

Given the modern fast-pass-through technology available for bioassay at the cellular and molecular level, continued sampling of marine and land based sources, including microorganisms, insects and arthropods, may still turn up an occasional highly useful compound that we missed for the want of today's much more powerful technology. The search should go on with the rapid microtechniques now available for finding even the most subtle molecular effects. Arthropod, amphibian, insect, and marine toxins, and growth control substances, most surely hold some priceless therapeutic surprises.

Final judgment about the actual clinical effectiveness of the Polynesian pharmacopoeia should not rest entirely on the classic screening technology of past decades. Renewed interest in alternative care continues to raise questions of efficacy that may well be answered by renewed efforts to rescreen these ethnopharmic materials with modern molecular technology.

CHAPTER 12

Some Drolleries

Along with our research activities, there always remained our primary raison d'etre, the treatment of our patients who were brought in by their friends by car, or on a plantation bus, which serviced the area, or in an ancient ambulance, which ran remarkably well with some prodding.

One day our ambulance went out to a distant house to pick up a lady who had suddenly started labor at home. Once the good lady was safely on board the ambulance stretcher, the driver and three men could not negotiate the corner of her hallway, so she calmly got up and walked out to the ambulance and climbed in—the baby appearing in this world then and there. Complicating matters, the ambulance was stuck in the mud, and after much expert advice from assembled neighbors, the whole works had to be towed out. Mother and baby did very well, and everyone enjoyed the unexpected entertainment.

Except for such surprises, hospital births were routine and occurred two or three times a week. Our patients prided themselves on accepting no anesthetic, and fortunately, our complications were few. Emergency surgeries were occasionally memorable occasions when things didn't quite go as planned. We did appendectomies, tubal ligations, hernia repairs, and a few tonsillectomies—all with open drop ether right from the can, with a safety pin through the little lead cap. It was a safe anesthetic as long as one included plenty of air and did not blow up the place.

We were lucky, and with a generally strong, healthy, well nourished population, we had few complications either in surgery or obstetrics. More difficult cases were referred to surgeons in Hilo, or Honolulu.

Our hospital and dispensary staff, usually permanent, locally born, on-the-job trained workers, was superb. Not everyone is attuned to rural life. Various lab techs, x-ray techs, and nurses came and went. Occasional characters that came from the mainland "to find themselves," often didn't.

One fine Christmas morning, a rather odd lady lab tech who occasionally helped in x-ray, and who was fresh from the mainland seeking romance in tropical paradise, suddenly packed her bags and stormed out of the hospital in a pyrotechnic rage, screaming, "He did it again; he did it again!" There was a small leak in the faucet that fed the x-ray film washing tank, and mysteriously, because of it, the water level in the tank would always rise during the night. Our paranoid lady was convinced that our x-ray man was "spiting" her by "pissing in the tank."

One temporary x-ray technician, of uncertain history and training, was having trouble with film exposures that were too dark or too light on several retakes. Finally, we found he thought 1/8 of a second was longer than 1/4, because eight is bigger than four. Cutting up a custard pie in the kitchen solved his problem in a tasty demonstration of mathematics.

Every child knows funny things happen in sets. Our set was already nicely launched with the ambulance baby, our lady lab tech, and the pie in the kitchen.

Our little run of oddities had one to go. A visiting executive from one of the state's larger landowning companies suffered a significant concussion, was unconscious, and had to be hospitalized for observation. All our hospital beds were full, with the exception of one in the labor room right next to the delivery table. We had many a later laugh with him over his astonishment on awakening, to find himself in the midst of a particularly messy delivery, not remembering his accident or admission to the hospital.

With humor, mutual respect, and a sense of timeless security, doctors and staff treasured the psychodynamics of our little medical enclave and its broad community support system. At the end of each year, when the huge mill engines were stopped, and the cane trucks ceased to rumble in the night, how proudly we celebrated, with workers and management, the joy of a bountiful sugar harvest. Oddly, we were only vaguely aware that jet travel, "big money," globalization, and the lure of greater profits from foreign agriculture, were quickly eating away at our hundred-year plantation culture and its doomed economy.

CHAPTER 13

Change

During the long period Hawaii's leaders spent in developing humane health care from the 1930s onward, creeping changes and competing interests were eroding the philosophy and funding of the entire system. Health insurance was born in the United States in 1930, nearly a half century after Otto Von-Bismarck introduced universal medical coverage to the German population. in 1884. This basic idea of medical insurance led in 1941 to trial runs of simple insurance plans for higher earners in the rural community of Kahuku on Oahu, and in Hawaii's capital city of Honolulu.

On this model, the Hawaiian Sugar Planters' Association, anticipating future cost rises, built a larger plan which it hoped "would continue to provide free doctor, nurse, and hospital facilities in spite of increased taxes, government, or labor demands. and should serve as a health cooperative for all the laborers, who would then pay for all the services they are now getting free." Proposed in 1940, the plan received a rejection, the first of many plan rejections for over 25 years.

By 1947, there was still no standardization of services. Each plantation provided facilities and care as it saw fit. Most had one or two salaried physicians, operated a dispensary offering unlimited diagnostic and outpatient services, ran or contracted with a conveniently located hospital, and provided supplementary health care such as field nurses and baby clinics. Workers and families resisted pressures for conversion to health insurance or to an independent prepaid program. The direct-service, plantation-managed, traditional program continued, while undergoing profound changes. Because of increasing costs and complexity of medical care, as well as the urbanization of rural areas and improved transportation, patterns of medical plan organization gradually shifted away from total company control. Aging plantation hospitals were retired in favor of new community hospitals, physicians moved into privately owned medical offices; where more and more physicians were paid through a variety of new contracts and fee schedules.

Cooperative arrangements developed between neighbor plantations for provision of dispensary services. In 1966, the non-profit Hamakua Infirmary Corporation, jointly controlled by four plantations at Honokaa, set an important example of this innovation, although each medical plan administration remained autonomous. By 1967 the product of this revolution was 25 separate plantation plans, sometimes partially coordinated, as in Honokaa. These used a bewildering variety of administrative methods, accounting procedures, and organization structures, despite a uniform benefit pattern based upon the industry-wide Union agreement of 1949. At that time the International Long Shore Workers' Union took its first step toward building the union's health and welfare program—the ILWU-PMA Welfare Plan. When the union and employers agreed to implement a disability insurance program in 1950, the plan was established and the first comprehensive package of medical, surgical, and hospital benefits went into effect.

A life insurance benefit was added mid-year, and in 1951 partial welfare coverage was extended to dependent family members, with full dependent coverage available in 1953.

The ILWU pioneered full hospital, medical, and surgical benefits for pensioners in 1952. In 1951, and again in 1961, the union initiated an unprecedented health-testing program for its long shore members as part of the larger concept of providing preventive health care.

During these many years of company-union disputes, the stable routines of dispensary and hospital care usually thrived in a calm born of distance from the negotiations, and dedication to patients. No one in a plantation community went untreated. As the plantations waned in wealth and influence, the dilemma then as now was how to continue this rare flowering of universal care.

By the time of full unionization, the 25 separate plantation medical plans were viewed as temporary, "awaiting an industry-wide permanent plan." Mainland consultants, as they left with their leis and boxes of pineapples, studiously agreed that we were all providing optimum care at minimum cost.

Finally, in 1954 a comprehensive medical plan agreement with the ILWU was signed which continued through 1967, providing full family care. This healthcare model was not limited to sugar plantations.

Pineapple Life

Plantation life in Hawaii's highly successful pineapple world closely reflects sugar's economic boom and "bust," its union history, its social organization and its universal healthcare plans. This socially successful culture is doomed to end with the picking of its last crop, planned for 2008.

In 1899, James Drummond Dole, a cousin of Sanford Dole, the first Territorial Governor of Hawaii, who had been deeply involved in American annexation, came from Harvard School of Agriculture to homestead in Hawaii. Pineapple plants were already here, brought by early ships. Dole dreamed of developing a vast world pineapple market. With only fifteen hundred dollars capital, he soon had land, and a cannery running, and had discovered the immense power of advertising. By 1923, he boasted that his crop, if extended as two parallel rows of plants, would run from New York to San Francisco, and that he had sold forty-four million cans of pineapple that year.

Part of his success may have sprung from his belief that "every employee may feel that his interest is that of the company, and vice versa." By 1939, ninety per cent of the world's pineapple lovers were enjoying Dole's Oahu shipments of canned pineapple, which included Lanai's 20,000-acre production.

Dole had about three thousand permanent, and seven thousand temporary workers. As with sugar production, mechanization and complex agricultural practices steadily boosted yields and greatly eased workers' labor in the fields..

Excellent houses and social services were provided, and universal medical care enhanced plantation life. As with the sugar industry, higher pay, and the amenities won by the ILWU after WWII, ensured steady production, but at progressively ruinous costs. The same economics that essentially ended the sugar world in Hawaii crushed the pineapple industry. Pineapples from low-wage countries are cheaper. Nothing else counts.

Dr. Paul Stevens, who has spent most of his professional life on Molokai, a small relatively undeveloped island near Oahu, has graciously provided an account of his early years in the pineapple world for this book. The engaging summary that follows highlights similarities in the changes that took place in the structure and operation of medical services for workers in the two plantation-based endeavors that dominated island life for so many years in the islands.

HEALTHCARE HAWAII STYLE

"Plantation Life on Molokai"
By Paul Stevens, M.D.

When I arrived on Molokai in 1956 to associate with Dr. Bill Totherow, the era of plantation medicine per se on Molokai, with the colorful and autonomous Plantation Doctor concept had pretty much faded away.

This happened in the early 50s when negotiations took place with management and the union (ILWU), and a contract was established with third party insurance carriers to bring about a health care program with free choice of physicians for employees and fee-for-service payments to the doctors. The doctors were from then on no longer fully paid by the companies as "Plantation Doctors." I believe this applied to the entire pineapple industry in Hawaii. However, the old concept didn't die instantly, and there were quite a few remnants which persisted and which we as private physicians were involved in.

In 1956 there were two active pineapple plantations on Molokai. Libby, McNeil was situated in Maunaloa on the west side of Molokai, and California Packing Corporation (later called Del Monte) was situated in Kualapuu in the central part of Molokai. Libby had previously had its own little hospital in Maunaloa as well as a company doctor and a company nurse.

Del Monte maintained a company nurse for several years until she retired in the sixties, and after that, they trained a personnel man to do the routine duties of the equivalent of a nurse's aide—screening sick employees, checking their blood pressures, and treating minor wounds. Anything more complicated. he would send down to our clinic.

On the other hand, Libby's nurse was a big old Polish gal who could handle almost anything. She ran the old Libby hospital and later maintained the Libby dispensary with an efficient and authoritative hand. She once told me that a lady came into her hospital one night and said she was about to deliver twins. Sally (the nurse) called the company doctor, who was at a party, and told him of the imminent delivery. He said, "Well go ahead and deliver her." She said, "I have never delivered twins!" and he said, "Neither have I. Go ahead and deliver her." So, she did, successfully.

I used to go up to the Libby Dispensary two or three times a week to hold an outpatient clinic. One day when I arrived, Sally was there with a cast on her arm. I said, "What happened to you?" She said, "I broke my arm over the weekend (Colles fracture), but I didn't want to bother you, so I set it myself and put on a cast." That was the typical kind of plantation nurse. They don't make 'em like that any more.

Although we were, by then, not employed or paid directly by the plantations, we were designated by management as the "preferred physicians" on the Island. We handled all of the workers' compensation cases, which in itself was often a can of worms. We had to act as not only the healer, but often as the policeman, when we had to determine whether or not a patient was malingering. Sometimes we had to try to get a patient back to work when the union was encouraging him to stay at home. The company, of course, was urging us to get him back to work, if possible.

As in Dr. Steven's practice, today, some fifty years later, industrial injury and illness authorities stress the value to patients and employers alike, of returning employees to work as soon as possible, at whatever level is appropriate, to reduce short and long term disability.

We did all the employee physicals once a year, usually about four or five hundred. We would show up at the company dispensary at 7:00 a.m. and do 10 or 20 physical examinations and then head to the hospital to make rounds, followed by a full day of office visits at our clinic. We, of course, delivered all of the babies, day and night. For a number of years, we did what was called "general practice surgery." This consisted of C-sections, appendectomies, herniorraphies, hysterectomies, vein strippings, gallbladders, even subtotal gastrectomies, and an occasional amputation. We also did upper GI series, barium enemas, cystoscopies, etc. This seems rather unusual in today's world, but in the days of the Plantation Doctor, it was considered routine.

We were expected to do everything. The alternative was to call in Hawaiian Airlines, have them remove some seats, install a stretcher, and ship the patient to Honolulu. To do that meant that there was something wrong with the doctor (incompetent?).

The hospital on Molokai was originally run by the Episcopal Church and called Shingle Memorial Hospital. In the early fifties the community took over the hospital and it became Molokai Community Hospital. The Board of Trustees was always heavily laced with plantation supervisors, so the needs of the employees were high on the hospital agenda. Around 1960, it was determined that the hospital was too decrepit to survive, so a fund drive was initiated to build a new facility. Every employee of the plantations contributed a percentage of his paycheck to this fund drive, and the new hospital was completed in 1963.

Dr. Stevens points out that at the time of his settling on Molokai, the plantations there were no longer paying physicians directly, but had involved third party payers. This did not affect physicians' services or the overall nature of care to workers and families since it was clearly understood that all patients would be seen regardless of the pay arrangements

As previously mentioned, we docs were not paid by the plantations, but we were given quite a few perks which were beneficial. Del Monte—had a "doctor's house," which was very spacious and rent was very cheap. We were given access to both the Libby golf course and the Del Monte golf course. Del Monte had access to a beach cottage on the North Shore, which was reserved for company supervisors, and the residing doctor was also given this privilege. The docs were always invited to all the company functions (translated parties), which may or may not have been considered a perk. (They were a "hard drinkin" bunch.)

In addition to the routine duties listed above, we were required to man the Emergency Room at the hospital 24 hours a day. Also, in those days it was considered part of the job to make house calls whenever requested, which always seemed to be at 2:00 or 3:00 a.m. This could mean going to the east end of the Island on a winding road or to the west end on an equally crooked road.

Most of our patients were Filipino or Japanese. Thank God for "Pidgin," which enabled us to communicate with those who were not too fluent in English. We learned to respect the ethnic customs, especially those that were related to various medical conditions. We found that it was not always appropriate to try to force Western medicine methods on patients who had been brought up with different beliefs.

Even today in the outlying areas of the islands, easy access to specialist care remains a problem. Honolulu clinics and hospitals have over the years arranged for traveling specialists who regularly see patients in the larger centers on the "outer islands," and one multispecialty Honolulu clinic provides full-time family practice care on Lanai. Dr. Stevens talks of some of the consultation issues he faced in early years:

One of the disadvantages of practicing on an isolated island was the lack of available specialists. Getting consultations by phone was nowhere nearly as effective as having the real person at the bedside. Over the years this tended to keep many potential doctors from locating on the Island. Getting adequate CME (continuing medical education) was always difficult. We had to rely mostly on medical audio tapes, occasional lectures from visiting specialists, and traveling off island to seminars.

Over the years, my relationship with the plantation managers was always very cordial. In fact, the manager of Del Monte was best man at my wedding. (Incidentally my spouse was a Queen's R.N. graduate whom I highjacked over to Molokai.) The manager of Libby Plantation, who was bought out by Dole around 1970, was a feisty guy who ruled with an iron hand but was a very effective manager and always very compatible with the local docs. Both plantations eventually closed down, Dole around 1977 and Del Monte in the late 1980s. The competition from foreign labor was too strong, and the need to transport the pineapples by barge to Honolulu became prohibitive. (Personal communication from Dr. Paul Stevens, 2 Jan. 2005).

CHAPTER 14

Connecting With The Larger World

On a delightful tropical island far from world troubles, traffic, stress, crime, and grinding competition, it is easy to ride one's personal waves of activity, closing the day with the adage painted on my first welcoming gift in Hawaii, one from our Kohala district local mom-and-pop store owner, Hideo Naito. It was a Japanese lacquered brown paper and bamboo umbrella sporting the words, "work finished is pleasant" on the four quadrants—so true, so focused, so pristine, and so ethnically exquisite. Amid this busy but peaceful world of plantation life, all the Honolulu hassle of union contracts, management meetings, payment and plan costs seemed others' vexations. Yet, in the end, connections with the larger world would gut the practice arrangements of most of our 45 physicians practicing on plantations in 1967, bringing benefit to some, and to others, just unsettling change.

The closing of plantation hospitals left doctors who were in private practice offices and dispensaries as the sole remnant of plantation care, except for the very welcomed scheduled visits by Honolulu-based consulting specialists whose arrival usually sparked a brief fishing trip or a jeep jaunt into the mountains, as well as a hard day's work.

Group Practice slowly became the norm. In 1961 four plantations near Hilo engaged Dr. William Bergin and four other physicians to form Hilo Clinic, to serve several plantations in a wide area. Three other partnership groups were established on Maui during the 1960s. This scenario repeated itself in all the larger population areas. This new structure for providing medical care favored centralization and prepayment.

By the late 1950s arrangements for care of plantation patients were common with insurance underwriters such as HMSA, the local "Blue Cross, Blue Shield" insurer which paid physicians specified fees for listed services.

In some areas, Kaiser Permanente Health Plans, which reached Hawaii from the mainland in 1958, became popular. Full family and multispecialty care is provided by salaried physicians working in Kaiser facilities. At this writing the Kaiser system operates nine clinics and an acute care hospital on Oahu, four clinics on Maui, and three on Hawaii island.

Many established physicians facing deep changes in their office economics chose to work under fee-for-service plans such as those of HMSA, which paid them by visit or procedure. However, the successes of the Kaiser plans have attracted many physicians to a salaried life. Fearful early warnings of creeping "socialized medicine" under the Kaiser plans are rarely heard today.

As health care costs rose everywhere, insurance contracts with HMSA and Kaiser health plans relieved to some extent, plantation companies' health care costs. Under the new arrangements, some of the burden of payment for services fell on employees and families enrolled through insurance plans that required patient co-payments to physicians and hospitals. In addition to insuring through third party payers such as HMSA, the large Oahu, Maui, and Kauai plantations arranged for their employees' care in centralized facilities, with the service improvements possible with a wider range of physician coverage, resources, equipment, and staffing.

What did universal health care for its workers cost the sugar industry in recent years? The dollar commitment of the Hawaiian sugar companies to full coverge has some value in present planning efforts to close the widening gap of uninsured in Hawaii and the nation. Here are some costs for the 1960s even when fees, hospital and drug costs were much lower than now.

Sugar Operations Only Medical Care Costs 24 Plantations		
Year	Percent of Gross Sugar Income	Percent of Net Sugar Income
1962	2.0	26.0
1963	1.8	15.9
1964	1.9	30.7
1965	2.0	29.3
1966	2.2	26.2
Average	1.9	25.6

From confidential records, "Recapitulation of Financial Information, 6/15/67"
Hawaii Agricultural Research Center, HSPA Library.

If one considers the net sugar income as comparable with the gross domestic product of the plantatiions, we find that the 25 percent healthcare outlay for full overage was far higher than the 15 percent said to be the fraction of national GDP paid out for medical care in the U.S.A. today. And today, economists predict a rise to that level for acceptable care. The substantial expenditures by Hawaiian sugar plantations in the 1960s showed a truly remarkable commitment, made of course, under significant union pressure. As sugar profits fell, the need to shift some of this cost burden to employees and the theoretical cost-controlling activities of insurers was clear. In the transition, elements were saved out of the old plantation plans, such as the strong public health features and facility mergers that largely preserved universal health care efforts in the state. Smaller communities in Hawaii successfully combined their medical resources in ways that were well outlined in the 1975 book *Humanizing Health Care*, by Dr. Robert Rushmer, who envisioned centralized facilities employing a broad spectrum of physicians and health care ancillaries in a nationwide system with a simplified payment source.

Many of Rushmer's recommendations have, in fact, been implemented in Hawaii, except for the single payer aspect. In Hawaii that disadvantage is partly offset by the overwhelming coverage by only three payers, Kaiser, HMSA, and Medicare/Medicaid.

Very successful mergers of scattered plantation hospitals were forged at Hilo, Hawaii, and Wailuku, Maui, and on the island of Kauai, with greatly expanded programs. Specialists living on outer islands and the provision of complex services marked the changes from simpler activities of earlier years. Most funding for actual services comes from private, county and state insurance plans, including HMSA, Kaiser, Medicare and Medicaid.

Major facilities, together with private offices, often as part of group practice, continue to serve plantation families and the many descendants of these families who now often have other sources of income or public assistance with which to pay. In short, we have in Hawaii inherited from the plantation system enviable care delivery over most of the state. Still it is with great concern in the first part of the twenty-first century that we watch our population falling into the same abyss of under, or non-insurance now plaguing the rest of the nation.

A few rural hospitals have continued to operate in remote areas such as Naalehu and Kohala on Hawaii. These, together with the larger centers, have been united administratively in a very successful organization that has enabled them to survive despite the economic problems facing them in caring for a largely low or no-income population. This remarkable entity is the

Hawaii Health Systems Corporation

The Hawaii Health Systems Corporation (HHSC) was established by Act 262, Session Laws of Hawaii 1996, as an agency of the State of Hawaii when it was given the responsibility of organizing Hawaii's state hospitals into an integrated system. The corporation retains the historical character of these hospitals in location, staffing and services offered, particularly those in rural areas, to preserve and enhance their relationships with the communities they serve in five regions across the state. HHSC is governed by a 13-member, voluntary Board of Directors responsible for developing policies, procedures, and rules necessary to plan, operate, and manage this complex and successful entity.

HHSC is a public benefit corporation of the State of Hawaii. As the State's community hospital system, HHSC fulfills the state's promise to provide quality "hometown" health care, particularly in the rural locations where private hospitals are unwilling or unable to provide services. HHSC is an essential part of our island community, on the same level as fire and police service. Although many mainland states have similar governance and support structures for their acute care hospitals, the Hawaii program is most remarkable for also providing long-term care services at reasonable rates, a benefit that has long existed in European plans, but is rare in the United States. In the provision of this service alone, Hawaii is a model for similar national coverage of the aged and chronically ill.

Today, the state of Hawaii has the fourth largest public hospital system in the U.S.; it is the fifth largest employer in Hawaii, and the largest provider of medical services for Hawaii's neighbor island population and visitors to the state. HHSC's current budget is close to $350 million, over ninety percent of which comes from corporation revenues for patient care. State support is approximately 6 percent; the balance is realized from outside sources such as grants and gifts. The system employs 3,400 employees to staff 1,260 beds on five islands.

CHAPTER 15

The Transition Beyond Plantation Medicine

In the 1970s, as the heyday of plantation life drew to a close, the forty-five or so physicians serving the workers and their families in plantation medical plans found themselves drifting off to other arrangements for further training, to join groups, to retire, or to stay in their districts as independent practitioners.

For me, in 1971, the opportunity came for more basic research in established laboratories, with the exciting development of the four-year medical school in Honolulu with its focus on family medicine, health care delivery systems and care access. All this led me, with the closing of Kohala Plantation, to an appointment to the Department of Physiology and to ten years of teaching and administration in the dean's office of the University of Hawaii School of Medicine, sending some seven hundred students for six-week preceptorships in the offices and clinics of fellow physicians for practical on-site experience locally and throughout Micronesia.

Most of these former students, now well into their practice years, recall with amusement those early weeks "out of the nest." One, then a nun, tells of doing her first delivery in an open boat in a nighttime crossing of a large Micronesian lagoon, her personal version of *"A Night To Remember."*

As the new John A. Burns School of Medicine in Honolulu blossomed in the late 1960s under the charismatic guidance
of Dean Dr. Terrence Rogers, a brilliant ex-potato farmer with
a Ph.D. in physiology and a WWII Royal Air Force bomber
background, the school's intent was to provide for effective primary care throughout the Pacific, through training our students
to provide affordable, competent care at every economic level.

Great concern for universal care access and public health
have alway been the hall-marks of Hawaii's schools of medicine
and public health. Major programs addressed the availability
and quality of care throughout Micronesia, with on-site training of indigenous health workers as far away as Yap and Palau.
Through Senator Daniel Inouye, federal funding of health programs enhanced community health centers that kept the state
of Hawaii a leader in health care availability in both rural and
city settings. Working at the School of Medicine within these
programs, and at Straub Clinic and Hospital, a multispecialty
physicians' group, it soon became clear to me that issues of disease and mortality rates, patient satisfaction, clinical outcomes,
medico-legal strife, and particularly, care access were for most
patients and areas of the state, better than in most mainland
states that reported up to 45% of their people medically uninsured. Why the difference? One reason is clear.

Hawaii's Unique Prepaid Healthcare Act

In 1974, Hawaii legislators passed the Prepaid Healthcare
Act, mandating health insurance for those working more than
20 hours a week. Union and government workers were exempt,
as unions negotiated coverage in their labor contracts. Hawaii is
the only state with such a law, heralded nationwide as a possible
way to minimize the number of uninsured.

New state licensing provisions for ancillary care professions, such as licensed nurse practitioners, have helped to reduce care costs, increasing first-level care coverage in government-supported health centers and private clinics and hospitals.

The New "Twenty Hour Work Week" in Hawaii—and two "unintended consequences."

Hawaii's state programs and mandatory employee coverage continued until recently to provide health services for over ninety percent of its population. As costs rose, reality struck employers who, under Hawaii's mandated health insurance laws, had no recourse but to reduce their benefits to survive. Now Hawaii's insured coverage has dropped to only 90 percent, wih a new unforeseen problem.

In an article by Maria Torres Kitamura in the December 2004 issue of *Hawaii Business*, Professor Gerard Russo of the University of Hawaii, Department of Economics, was quoted as saying "New research confirms that Hawaii's mandated health insurance law has led to fewer work hours for part-timers."

The Prepaid Healthcare Act has apparently encouraged Hawaii employers to hold down part-time work hours compared to the rest of the nation. Professor Russo also said,"We have a lot of stories about employers not hiring people full-time because they have then to provide health insurance. It is not completely changing the economy, but the data seem to indicate that there is an effect." By requiring employers to provide benefits to employees who work 20 hours a week he says "the Prepaid Health Care Act has, in practice, changed the definition of full-time work in Hawaii."

Despite these deterrents, employer-based plans will surely predominate unless a national plan evolves.

Toward Universal Health Care

Hawaii's medical care history is indeed complex and unique.

Hawaii's culture, aspirations, industries and government have evolved one of the most complete care systems in the country, Is this the sort of coverage the nation wants, and how would it like to pay for it?

Some recent excerpts from the November 2004 issue of *Issue Briefs, a publication of the Employee Benefits Research Institute in Washington, D.C. quoted* by R. Helman, Greenwald Associates, reveal much about what Americans really want from their health insurance and how they want to pay for it. Over 20 percent of those contacted consider health care the most critical issue facing the country, ranking ahead of the economy, the war, education, the budget deficit, and terrorism.

Respondents are greatly disturbed by health care costs, the premiums, co-pay payments, and drugs. Access to care, the availability of needed treatment, and the uncertainty of future care, all simply mirror the difficulty in many areas of finding a sympathetic, available physician for office and hospital care at a reasonable price. Those with household incomes less than $70,000 a year feel especially vulnerable. Those with government plans are more satisfied than those with employer-based plans. Other proposals such as Health Savings Accounts and tax benefit schemes rank last.

Nearly half of those surveyed, even the insured, report going to the doctor only as a last resort. Many switched to alternative medicine practitioners or over-the-counter drugs, actions largely cost driven. More than half of the respondents felt they could not find or pay for insurance if they were given the money paid out by employers for health coverage, **clearly indicating preference for employer-sponsored plans.** Confidence in Medicare, which has been remarkably successful, is waning as the current U. S. presidential administration threatens to undermine its provisions with Alice in Wonderland "improvements." .

Remarkably, while more insured Americans are dissatisfied with their current health care than in the past, many are not eager to switch to any new plan that assigns them more responsibility for their care, especially if it increases their costs. Despite the fact that more than half of Americans agree that direct involvement in their treatment decisions would improve their care, 67 percent of these do not seek or welcome this responsibility for making decisions. When queried further, their response was, "When you go to the doctor, you simply follow the advice." Confidence in physicians is still high, but confidence in much of the health care insurance market place is not. Patients cherish the power of their employers to maximize benefits in health plan negotiations and to act as a buffer against greedy insurers.

Employee benefits are of primary importance to eight in ten Americans when choosing a job. A fourth of the working population would welcome better coverage, even at the cost of some income, if provided through the employer. These views, generated by what appears to be a valid study, point to a yearning among American workers and families for a stable, employer-based system.

More Expert Opinions About Care Access and Payment

In 1992, Emily Friedman, an independent writer, lecturer, and health policy and ethics analyst presently based in Chicago, Ill., focused her attention on Hawaii's health care history and status in *The Aloha Way: Health Care Structure and Finance in Hawaii*, a Hawaii Medical Service Association Foundation publication.

As the contributing editor of *Hospitals and Health Networks* and contributing writer for the *Journal of the American Medical Association, Health Progress,* and other periodicals, noted for her work in health policy, health care trends, social ethics of managed care, and health care for the underserved, her analysis of Hawaii's remarkably broad insurance coverage, the social factors involved, and how they might relate to development of a better national universal health care system, is trenchant.

Before considering her proposals of how Hawaii's health plans might point to national solutions for distribution and payment for health services, here are some of her views on American health care, published in the Winter 2003 issue of *Health Forum Journal*.

"Death Spiral"
By Emily Friedman

"The fact that more than 41 million Americans are uninsured provokes studies, commissions, debates, hand-wringing and buck-passing. Why don't we act?

It has become a rather sad autumn ritual. Every September, the Census Bureau announces how many Americans had no health insurance the previous year. The announcements produce the usual responses, ranging from a demand for a single-payer system from the Left to a shrug from the Right.

It's not like this is a recently discovered problem. The agency then known as the National Center for Health Services Research (now the Agency for Healthcare Research and Quality) in 1978 issued the pioneering report that counted 26 million people without coverage. That was followed up by study after study after study, each carefully documenting the rise in the number of uninsured Americans, often with detailed data about their race, gender, age and location."

Ms. Friedman further cites the findings of the Institute of Medicine, a branch of the National Academies of Sciences, organized under Congressional charter, consisting of twelve hundred of the world's public health experts appointed through peer review:

According to the Institute of Medicine (IOM), 18,000 Americans die each year as a direct result of lacking insurance. And that figure does not include all those who die further down the line because of undiagnosed (or, worse yet, diagnosed but untreated) hypertension, diabetes, heart disease, AIDS, cancer and other serious conditions. And those physicians, hospi-

tals and clinics that continue to provide care to as many of the indigent as possible are drowning in oceans of red ink. In more than one instance, it has cost the hospital its life [twenty three acute care general hospitals in California closed through financial failure in 1995 through 2000].

Employers, traditionally, have been the source of most private insurance, and for the most part they have tried to stay the course. But they are feeling the pressure from double-digit health care cost inflation, the rising prices of prescription drugs and hospital services and skyrocketing premiums to afford it."

In 2005 the average premium for reasonably good medical coverage for a family of four was approximately eleven thousand dollars, and the percentage of the Gross Domestic Product was 16 percent, considerably more than in other developed countries. Health care costs in the United States have risen to a level that employers alone can no longer fund without help from either co-pay by patients, or government-based assistance, leaving some 45 million persons uninsured. Ms. Friedman explains why nothing is done at the Federal level about these unfortunates.

"The Excuse"
By Emily Friedman

"First, the uninsured are disproportionately poor, and minority groups are at much higher risk. To ignore the racial discrimination implicit in this whole matter is to be naïve.

Second, we face a difficult ideological split. The Bush administration has proposed tax credits for the uninsured, an approach supported by most Republicans in both houses of Congress. Although it is an appealing approach theoretically, it is rooted more in a private-sector-above-all mentality than in reality.

Those who want a public program, whether a single-payer or largely expanded Medicaid, Medicare, State Children's Health Insurance Program (SCHIP) or other initiative, seem to be blissfully ignorant of the fact that the amount of taxpayer money involved would be very large indeed. They are equally unaware, apparently, of the kind of battle this nation would get into if we decided to nationalize the private insurance industry."

Despite this warning, individual states and the media appear to be wooing some sort of universal coverage. Health economists argue about whether insurance should be a government or private enterprise, mandatory or voluntary, perhaps with a single payer as in Canada or New Zealand. The lobbying pressure of competing players such as the present insurance giants, the American Medical Association, the ARRP, and hospital interests vastly complicate planning. Definitions matter. For example, "single-party payer" and a "salaried practice" should not be lumped together with a vague "nationalized practice" hysteria.

The most organized approach at the national level is the proposal of the Physicians for a National Health Care Plan (PNHP), a 14,000-member group based in Cambridge, Mass., that proposes a National universal tax based single-payer plan. Its members, with avid supporters in every state, believe such a system in inevitable. While most hospitals and clinics would remain privately owned and operated, the federal health care entity would control the purse strings, setting a monthly budget for the facilities' operating costs and paying them no more than the budget allowed. Investor-owned facilities would be converted to non-profit status and private insurance companies would essentially be eliminated. Strong contrary opinions exist.

Violently opposed to the single-payer aspect of this plan are many members of the American Medical Association, whose spokesman, and past president, Dr. Donald Palmisano, has said in many addresses around the country, that the plan " would lead to long lines, an even thicker health-care bureaucracy, and a slowness to adopt new technologies and maintain facilities."He has warned against turning health care over to the government, emphasizing the essential role the private sector plays in health care. "Private industry, not the government, has led the way in adopting disease management programs and prescription drug coverage. Innovation almost always begins in the private sector. It is very difficult for the government to innovate and change with changing times."

Linda Gorman, of the Rocky Mountain Center for Health Care Policy, agrees with Dr. Palmisano that the single-payer approach seriously threatens the quality of health care and positive medical outcomes that currently set U.S. health care apart from the rest of the world.

"The poor performance of single-payer systems can be seen in cancer mortality ratios, the death rate divided by the incidence of disease, she writes. *For breast cancer, the U.S. mortality ratio is 25 percent. In Canada and Australia it is 28 percent, in Germany it is 31 percent, in France it is 35 percent, and in New Zealand and the United Kingdom it is 46 percent. For prostate cancer, the U.S. mortality ratio is 19 percent. In Canada it is 25 percent, in New Zealand it is 30 percent, in Australia it is 35 percent, in Germany it is 44 percent, in France it is 49 percent, and in the United Kingdom it is 57 percent."* (Denver Post, Road to Medical Hell, 11 Jan 03, pEI). **Factors other than method of payment could well cause these differences and have nothing to do with single-payer provisions.**

Another expert, Greg Scandlen, director of the Center for Consumer Driven Health Care at the Galen Institute, a health and tax policy research organization in Alexandria, Va., has said on various occasions that countries that adopted the [single payer] approach are racing to change it. And while Americans are registering discontent with the health care status quo, Scandlen points to surveys by Dr. Robert Blendon of Harvard University that show a similar level of discontent among the people of Canada, the United Kingdom, Australia, and New Zealand wherein popular support (for single-payer health care) in Canada has plunged in the past 10 years. These countries now see that a single-payer approach leads to rationed care, high rates of taxation, and the virtual banishment of new technology and innovation.

Greg Scandlen confirmed his views on single-payer systems in a letter to me dated July 2006, saying:

The only true Single Payer system left in the world is Canada, and perhaps Cuba. Everywhere else it is possible, even expected, that people will go outside the government system to purchase some of their health care needs. The UK, for instance, has a thriving and growing private health insurance industry. With the recent (June 2005) Supreme Court decision in Canada, [permitting purchase of care outside the nationalized system] even that country's Single Payer system is in jeopardy.

Clearly from these quotations, there is great angst among care providers about quality and adequate financial support for a universal health care system, particularly with a single party payer. Emily Friedman says that *the only approach that has a prayer of working is "some kind of hybrid involving public subsidy of private coverage in a market that is heavily regulated to prevent the picking off of good risks, and the avoidance of bad risks.*

Medical insurance in Hawaii, with two major commercial plans and significant state support for the indigent largely meets these goals, although fee-for-service payment levels to private physicians and hospitals are continually in dispute.

Doing Nothing

Emily Friedman has concerns other than methods of payment. *In some settings on the mainland, there are those who like the status quo 'just fine.' There is no subtle way to say this. Even beyond the ideology, which is pretty fierce, there are proposals and policies that cannot be explained other than by assuming that there are interests who don't want the problem addressed; they just want it to go away.*

Perhaps the worst example of this is the new federal Health Insurance Flexibility and Accountability Initiative (HIFA), through which the Bush administration is granting waivers to states to provide "insurance" to those who are uninsured and ineligible for other programs. For many, their insurance will be worthless. Here is an example.

Dr, Friedman tells of the Idaho Legislature, which for two years in a row zeroed out all funds for outreach for the state's Child Health Insurance Program and Medicaid because, in the words of one legislator, "we are signing up too many children." She says further:

> *As long as policy-makers see the uninsured as powerless and therefore un-likely sources of campaign contributions (which is, unfortunately, largely true), as long as bigots see people of color as less deserving than themselves, as long as the insured are more worried about getting coverage for cosmetic surgery than about those who are dying of treatable cancers, as long as providers are just as glad not to have to bother with "those" people, and as long as the uninsured are 'them' and not 'us,' then the status quo will hold.*

Many obcess over the nagging question of whether proper care should be considered a "right" or simply a marketable commodity like food, entertainment, or laundry soap.

Unfortunately it is true in the United States that realistic legislative interest in providing care for the indigent is at the bottom of the priority barrel. One of Emily Friedman's European friends said to her, "it doesn't matter if you have such good care if people cannot have access to it." True insight. Friedman believes that *"sooner or later we will do something. But only after tens of thousands more people have died, and only after many good, conscientious health* *care organizations have gone up the flume because they cared, and only after insurance providers who avoid the uninsured have gone home laughing with their millions. This doesn't have to happen. We can force the issue. We can stop being polite, and being afraid to offend anyone, and being unwilling to make trouble, and being able to tolerate the slow torture and killing of our neighbors. We can stop this. **The question, in the end, is whether we want to.**"*

Dr. Friedman's questions cut directly to morality, ethics, and distributive justice. All of us, patients, care providers, investors, planners, and lawmakers, live in a stew of conflicting motivations, which block the course to universally available care. Plans to date founder mainly on issues of power and profit.

CHAPTER 16

A Healthy Try That Ran Amok

Another convincing national leader is President Bill Clinton, who in his address to congress in 1993 summarized the problems and possible solutions. That all this was shot down politically is history, but a history that has, by inaction, brought catastrophe to countless homes, hospitals, and many of the lives of 45 million uninsured Americans.

In President Clinton's address, he specifically mentioned Hawaii's remarkable access to quality health services His observations on what might be done for the nation as a whole are still valid today, some fourteen years later:

"Despite the dedication of literally millions of talented health care professionals, our health care is too uncertain and too expensive, too bureaucratic and too wasteful. It has too much fraud and too much greed.

First and most importantly [we need] security. Security means that those who do not now have health care coverage will have it, and for those who have it, it will never be taken away. Programs would provide a broad range of preventive services including regular checkups and well-baby visits.

We must maintain the Medicare program. It works to provide that kind of security. Medicare should provide coverage for the cost of prescription drugs."

Recent Federal legislation attempts such as the 2003 Medicare Part D to address this issue; is at best controversial, and may well be a financial disaster for middle-income patients.

Over time, we should phase in long-term care for the disabled and the elderly on a comprehensive basis. The most rapidly growing percentage of Americans is those over 80. We cannot break faith with them.

The second principle is simplicity. Our health care system must be simpler for the patients and simpler for those who actually deliver health care. Today we have more than 1,500 insurers requiring the completion of hundreds and hundreds of different forms. These forms are time consuming, they're expensive for health care consumers, and they're exasperating for anyone who's ever tried to sit down around a table and wade through them and figure them out.

The medical care industry is literally drowning in paperwork. In recent years, the number of administrators in our hospitals has grown by four times the rate that the number of doctors has grown.

We want to let market forces enable plans to compete.

Unless everybody is covered, we will never be able to fully put the brakes on health care inflation. Without health insurance, people still get health care, but they get it when it's too late, when it's too expensive, often from the most expensive place of all, the emergency room.

We have to crack down on fraud and abuse. (This has been widely addressed through the Office of the Inspector General and compliance legislation.) *Large savings have been achieved. These could be used to cover the unemployed uninsured.*

President Clinton then discussed companies and states that have held down premiums, mentioning Hawaii as the only state that covers virtually all of our citizens and has still been able to keep costs below the national average.

Free choice is important. We propose to give every American, each year, a choice among high-quality plans. (This is mandated in Hawaii.) *You can stay with your current doctor, join a network of doctors and hospitals, or join a health maintenance organization.*

Quality is something that we simply can't leave to chance. When you board an airplane, you feel better knowing that the plane had to meet standards designed to protect your safety. And we can't ask any less of our health care system. A sound system will create reports on health plan quality.

Quality reporting systems are in now in place in many states, with Internet disclosure of standings. Quality reports for USA hospitals can be found on line at <http://www.qualitycheck.org/index.htm>

High quality medical information must be available in even the most remote areas of this country, linking rural doctors, for example, with hospitals with high-tech urban medical centers. Drug charges should not be larger than (those) overseas.

President Clinton then discussed the need for personal responsibility for life style issues—to lessen the burden on health care of violence, drugs and alcohol, and for obesity with its complications. He then said:

I believe that all of us should have insurance and that most of the money would come from employers and workers' compensation. Why should the rest of us pick up the tab when a guy who doesn't think he needs insurance or says he can't afford it gets in an accident, winds up in an emergency room, gets good care, and everybody else pays?

Most of the money will come from premiums paid by employers and individuals Some call it an employer mandate, but I think it's the fairest way to achieve responsibility in the health care system. Every employer should provide coverage, just as three-quarters of them do now.

Over the long run, we can all win. This is our chance. This is our journey. And when our work is done, we will know that we have answered the call of history and met the challenge of our time.

We have not met the challenge of our time. The task remains as our health services crumble.

CHAPTER 17

More Critical Insights

On 17 January 2004, a brilliant summary appeared in *The Economist*, a highly respected British news publication. It discussed health care delivery issues in developed countries, presenting facts that could assist in U.S. planning, but only if there is public and honest political support for change. We have seen in *Helman's Briefs* (pg. 138) a slice of the American view of what is needed. Here are some further ideas from *The Economist* article, *The Health of Nations, p.3.*

> *In America, publicly financed health care goes mainly to the old and the poor; most workers and their families are insured privately through their employers. During much of the 90s, the cost of these employer-funded benefits has been rising. Alain Beethoven, a health economist at Stanford University who has pioneered cost-control strategies, paints a scenario in which continuing cost explosion opens the door for a government takeover of employer financed health care after the 2008 presidential election.*

According to the article, Dr. Beethoven suggests that employer financed health care plans should give way to a tax-based system funding hospitals and physicians' services for all, despite the brewing dissatisfaction voiced by Canadians with their tax-based system.

What is Life Worth? Extended life as a commodity.

Health care spending by rich nations such as Great Britain, Germany, and France averages about 10 percent per year of their of their gross domestic product and is rising. The United States average is about 15 percent. This may very well be a bargain. Detailed research in cardiovascular disease, and similarly in metabolic and infectious disorders, suggests the benefits of such spending greatly exceed the costs, and the money is well spent. Simply put, many of us are simply buying time—buying days, weeks, months and years of life. It can be expensive, and if chosen and paid for, will certainly change our spending habits.

Some sound reasons for rising health costs and why one might even welcome them are suggested by four of *The Economist's* commentators:

New technologies demand more health workers—hospitals are labor intensive, accounting for more than 60 percent of American hospital expenses. William Bauman, an economist at New York University says health care is "a handicraft industry" afflicted by the chronic "cost disease of personal services."

Technology may be raising costs, but only because the market is ready to pay for expensive innovations. So, what is life worth?

Here are some further suggestions from *The Economist* review:

Until recently, most health economists were skeptical about the contribution of medical care to general health, says Dr. Ted French of University of California, Santa Barbara. A former skeptic himself (about the economic effects of health care) *he now argues that even allowing for the effect of lifestyles, medical care does make a difference. He is convinced about the value of drugs, especially the cholesterol-lowering statins used to counter cardiovascular disease. His analysis of 18 advanced countries suggests that pill-popping does work, saying that countries that consumed more pharmaceuticals saw their populations live longer and suffer less ill health than those that consumed less.*

Why we are Looking at 15-to-30 Percent of GNP for Health Care

William Schwartz of the University of California School of Medicine stresses that medical care delivers more than longer lives through greater mobility, enhanced vision and pain relief, and that the cost of such treatment accounts for much of the spending gap between America and other countries. In a recent book, *"Your Money or Your Life"* David Cutler, an economist at Harvard University, says an American, aged 45 today will live four and a half years longer than in 1950 because of better medical care and related behavioral changes.

Mr. Cutler estimates that an extra year of life is worth $100,000 to an individual. To most individuals in reasonable health, life is priceless. **He suggests that it may be entirely reasonable to accept even the expenditure of 30 percent of GNP as the value and price of our longevity and health.**

With these suggestions that the purchase of life and health will richly justify the future spending of larger percentages of the gross national product for health care, we will be seeing an even larger portion of discretionary income going into medical care—inevitable if people truly want prompt access to "miracle" drugs and procedures.

An often ignored fact in healthcare discussions is that healthcare is a significant part of our GNP, that provides the daily living and economic security of hundreds of thousands of productive workers and entities at every level. These payments stay almost entirely within the country. What is wrong about the increase in a portion of the GNP that delivers highly esteemed services and products that increase lifespan and quality of life? To pay for these improvements, premiums are rising; co-pay is becoming more common and sizeable. Cash-up-front stand-alone facilities are blossoming, and we may well be on course for a two-tiered system with appropriate payment for both plans, like those emerging in the present National Health programs of Great Britain, Canada, and Germany.

Some Cost Savings May Be Possible

While health care costs will almost certainly consume more and more discretionary income, a direct attack on unnecessary costs comes from Dr. Don Berwick, President and Chief Executive Officer of the Institute for Health Care Improvement in Boston, Massachusetts. Dr. Berwick, with convincing data since 1998 holds that care in the USA has serious faults that result in enormous preventable losses through unwarranted procedures, errors, morbidity, and death. Based on clinical evidence, he proposes these six simple hospital care changes that have begun to save lives and money:

1. Provide rapid response teams for the critically ill.
2. Base heart attack care on statistically proven data.
3. Develop standardized care methods for patients on ventilators, to prevent pneumonias.
4. Develop standardized care methods for patients with central catheters, to prevent infection.
5. Use preoperative antibiotics to prevent surgical infections.
6. Develop standard plans to monitor and coordinate patients' medications.

These rational attempts to cut costs will not alone save our hospitals or care quality. Adequate federal healthcare payments to states appear to be doomed. Budget cuts, unfunded mandates such as free emergency department services for non-paying patients, low or non-payment for complex expensive procedures, and draconian billing requirements, are causing hospital failures across the nation. Overwhelming political action is needed **now** to wake up complacent bureaucrats that dither while care quality crumbles.

Until recently, care access has been available for ninety five per cent of Hawaii's population—the result of strong union pressure, reasonable Federal support, and the cultural and historic expectations of its people. Credit for this success must also be given to employers, to our largest and relatively efficient insurers, HMSA and Kaiser, our state hospital system, and to the physicians who continue to work in this shrinking financial milieu.

Budding systems, Take Note—

In 1992, Emily Friedman wrote: *Several major lessons can be gleaned from the Hawaii experience to date, as well as numerous minor ones. Perhaps the most important is that near-universal coverage can be achieved without collapsing a state's economy or driving all employees and payers out of business. Amiable political relationships and strong leaders bring concensus.* Universal access is much more difficult if you try to do it all at once. A start with employers can be followed up with programs targeted to those still left out of the system.

Here is how to build a successful universal care program at the state level:

1. Make preventive and primary care a high priority. Hawaii's plantations did this; preventive services were real, with impressive results

2. Stress collaborative policy making. There was an underlying vein of cooperation in forging policy in Ha-

waii, in which insurers, employers, hospitals, physicians, and government all contributed to the success. There is simply an understanding that at times it is necessary to check the guns at the door.

3. Address basic needs. Proper housing, social services, and nutrition underlie health care.

4. Stress cost containment. If private insurers are involved, they must be non-profit with minimal overhead.

5. Control insurers. They must not compete to avoid risks, thus cutting the sick out of the system. A strong Insurance Commission is essential.

For the present, multiple-payer plans can work, and are much closer to acceptability than a single-payer system. At the time of this writing, two states, Massachusetts and Vermont have passed laws mandating universal care. It will be tax-financed for low earners and the indigent, buttressed by private insurance and employee contributions. Both plans, scheduled to start in 2007 insure every state resident (ARRP Bull.July/Aug 06, pg. 99). As with Hawaii's coverage, neither is a single-payer plan. California has joined the movement and similar new legislation is reported almost monthly, across the nation. Universal health care appears to be on the march in a multipayer mode.

CHAPTER 18

Who Pays, and How

This march of American states in moving, as Hawaii did long ago, to universal care with multiple funding sources—taxes, employer and employee contributions, copay and deductables, involes multiple payers to physicians, hospitals, and other care providers. Despite some computer relief, this means we must still endure swarms of paperwork—bills, billing rejections, receipts, and forms that may add as much as one third to medical care costs in wasted time and staffing needs in dealing with multiple payers.The way to end this waste is to operate under a single payer, urged by the Physicians for a National Health Program, a nationwide fourteen thousand member organization, other health care professionals, and political leaders. All these are pressing for a single-payer program wherein the government fully finances health care, but keeps the actual delivery of care under private control. This is the optimum solution for the United States, for both complete coverage and cost. The program should operate under non-governmental professional guidance, as seen with the Federal Reserve banking system. Its leadership must be leading physicians, public health experts, and economists. Members of the National Academy of Medicine would be a good start, working with members of other professions and citizen groups.

Twenty-eight industrial nations have single-payer universal health care systems. Most have been fully tax-supported for decades without causing a national crisis. Ultimate movement toward a universal single-party pay plan in the U. S. will certainly follow the present effort of states to provide full care through taxes, employer, and employee contribution if these models fail.

CHAPTER 19

Some Afterthoughts

Tonight as twilight falls over the vast ocean that influences the lives of all of us in Hawaii, I stand in our condominium garden, remote from the construction cranes and traffic outside, fascinated as always, by the rain-patter on the huge leaves dripping in our grove of Heliconia plants. Somehow, the sound of the steady rain and earthy odor of the garden inexplicably touch the thread that takes me back fifty years to the plantation and my injured Kohala dog who enjoyed the benefits of surgery in our little wooden hospital. Of course, the dog is long gone, as is the hospital—but the timeless spirit of the setting and the people to whom it often meant life and death remains, and I am awed by the continuity of it all.

From seeing my first real patients in my training days, the GIs in our wartime European hospital, the Wisconsin farm people in their bitter winter snows, Northwest fishermen and loggers in Bellingham, Washington, Nigerian jungle dwellers, and the Pacific Islanders on far-off atolls—all of those sick, injured, or worried whom I have known as my patients had one wish—to be helped NOW, if possible, with compassion, competence, and consideration of cost. This primal plea is not being met for everyone. This must change if we are to remain a cherished profession and not a crass business.

Even reasonably good health care systems in the United States are increasingly fragile. There are good and bad reasons for rising medical costs. State of the art devices and drugs are expensive, but are truly a bargain. Unacceptable costs—greedy insurers, excessive tort issues, and unrealistic lifestyle aspirations of a few physicians—these can be controlled. With the will to do it, we can limit the excesses in the way the Public Utility Commission controls gas, communication, and electricity prices. Realistic insurance coverage and rates, whether government or private, simplification of payment, relief from outrageous legal threat in daily practice, and adequate tax support of the truly indigent could produce a national health system that is workable.

It is time that the people of America demand this. The time has come for action. Write, call, email or visit your legislators—individually or through the power of organizations, to get moving on our primitive system. Give your lawmakers no peace until they have in place state or federal support for basic medical care for everyone. Slavery ended by public demand, civil rights came by the same route. National health coverage, with your help, will be next. Make your voice heard, **now.**

BIBILIOGRAPHY

1. Dorrence, William H.; Morgan, Francis S. Sugar Islands. Honolulu, Hawaii: Mutual Publishing; 2000. 259 p.

2. Takaki, Ronald. Pau Hana. Honolulu, Hawaii: University of Hawaii Press; 1983. 213 p.

3. Greer, Richard. In the Shadow of Death. Hawaii Historical Review, Selected Readings. Hong Kong, Cathay Press; 1969. p. 37-88.

4. Lewis, Francis R. Hegglund. History of Nursing in Hawaii. Node, Wyoming. Germann-Kilmer Co.; 1969. 135 p.

5. Cooper, G; Dawes, G. Land and Power in Hawaii. Honolulu, Hawaii. Benchmark Books; 1985. 518 p.

6. Dawes, G. Shoal of Time. Honolulu, Hawaii: University of Hawaii Press; 1968. 694 p.

7. Akana, A.; Akina, J. K. Native Hawaiian Medicines (Hawaiian Herbs) Chun, M. N.: translator and editor. Honolulu, Hawaii: First People's Productions; 1944. 276p.

8.	University of Hawaii, School of Medicine, Department of Pharmacology. Terminal Progress Report, Natural Products of the Pacific: PHS Grant GM 15198-01-03. Honolulu, Hawaii. 1972. 27 p. See as Appendix, page 108.

9.	James, J. Health Plan for Hawaii, (HSPA files). Honolulu, Hawaii. 1968. 27 p. Hawaii Agricultural Research Center.

***

These excerpts are from the bibliography compiled by JoAnn Tsark and Kim Birnie *Native Hawaiian Healthcre*, http:IIwww.nativehawaiianhealth.net/moku/indigenouspeople.cfm #

Abbott, Isabella. 1992. La'au Hawai'i; Traditional Hawaiian Uses of Plants, Honolulu: Bishop Museum Press.

Abbott, Isabella & Shimazu C. 1985. The geographic origin of the plants most commonly used for medicine by Hawaiians. Journal of Ethnopharmacology Nov-Dec;14(2-3):213-22.

Aiu, Patrick K. H. 1994 . Health Care Aboard the Hokulea Energy Requirement Study. Hawai'i Medical Journal 53: 352-353.

Akana, A, Akina JK, Ka'aiamanu DM. 1922. Hawaiian Herbs of Medical Value. Honolulu: Territorial Board of Health Bulletin.

Aluli, Noa Emmett. 1991. Prevalence of obesity in a Native Hawaiian population. American Journal of Clinical Nutrition Jun;53(6 Suppl): 1556S-1560S.

Aluli, NE. 1999. Hali'a Aloha'e Dr. Thomas Whelan. Hawai'i Medical Journal 58(11).

Andrade, Naleen & Noda, Kaoru. 1977. The incidence of intestinal parasites in some Hilo Hospital patients Hawai'i Medical Journal 36(6). sctivity. Molecular and Cellular Biology 19(3): 2338-2350.

Asian American and Pacific Islander Health Promotion (AAPIHP). 1997. Proceedings of "Cancer Crisis Among Asian Pacific Islanders as Articulated by Asian Pacific Islanders," Asian American and Pacific Islander Journal of Health 5. Head Neck Surg 117: 390-395.

Banner, Richard; DeCambra, Hooipo; Enos, Rachelle; Gotay, Carolyn; Hammond, Ormond; Hedlund, N; Issell, Brian; Matsunaga, Doris & Tsark JA. 1995. A breast and cervical cancer project in a Native Hawaiian community: Wai'anae Cancer Research Project. Preventive Medicine Sep;24(5): 447-53.

Baruffi, Gigliola; Sylva, Summer & Look, Mele. 1998. Health of Hawaiian women. Pacific Health Dialog 5(2): 290-6.

Beddow, Ralph & Arakaki, Richard. 1997. Non-Insulin Dependent Diabetes Mellitus: An Epidemic Among Hawaiians. Hawai'i Medical Journal 56.

Birnie KK. 1998. Cancer and Culture. Asian American and Pacific Islander Journal of Health 6(2): 382.

Birnie KK. 1998. Native Hawaiian Health Summit., Ke Ola Kino, Hawai'i Public Health Association newsletter: Spring 1998.

Blaisdell, Richard Kekuni. 1982. History of Medicine in Hawai'i. University of Hawai'i, Department of Medicine: 1982 (an outline).

Blaisdell RK. 1989. Historical and cultural aspects of Hawaiian health. In Social Process in Hawai'i, The Health of Native Hawaiians: A Selective Report on Health Status and Health Care in the 1980s, ed. EL Wegner, 32: 1-21., Honolulu: University of Hawai'i Press.

Blaisdell RK. 1993. The Health Status of Kanaka Maoli (Indigenous Hawaiians). Asian American and Pacific Islander Journal of Health, Autumn 1993 1(2):116-160.

Blaisdell RK. 1996. Update on Kanaka Maoli (indigenous Hawaiian) Health, Asian American and Pacific Islander Journal of Health, Winter-Summer 4(1-3):160-5.

Blaisdell RK. 1998. Cancer and culture in Kanaka Maoli (Native Hawaiians). Asian American and Pacific Islander Journal of Health 6(2): 400.

Boyd, Charles; Maunakea, Alika; Mordan, LJ & Csiszar, K. 1998. Polynesian ethnobotanicals: a critical role in new drug discovery. Pacific Health Dialog 5(2): 337-340.

Braun, Kathryn; Look, Mele & Tsark, Jo Ann. 1995. High mortality rates in Native Hawaiians. Hawaii Medical Journal Sep;24(5): 447-53.

Burgess, Lawrence P, Hessel CR. 1990. Software for logging of surgical cases. Otolaryngol Head Neck Surg 102: 145-149.

Arch Otolaryngol Head Neck Surg 119: 173-177.

Burton DM, Burgess LP. 1990. Nocardiosis of the upper aerodigestive tract. Ear Nose Throat J 69: 350-353.

Chang Healani. 1999. M_lama Ola Hawai'i (Hawaiian Health Care): an assessment of Hawaiian Healing Strategies. Dissertation submitted to University of Hawai'i at M_noa, Honolulu, Hawai'i.

Chong, Clayton DK; Aluli NE; Reyes Phillip W. 1999. Issues Affecting the Health of Hawaiians. Conference sponsored by the Native Hawaiian Center of Excellence, Hawai'i.

Chun, Malcolm (translator). 1986. Hawaiian Medicine Book-He Buke Laau Lapaau, Honolulu: Bess Press.

Chun, Malcolm (translator). 1994,1998. Native Hawaiian Medicine Volumes 1 and 2, Honolulu: First People's Productions.

Cockett, Abraham T & Ken Koshiba. 1996. Color Atlas of Urologic Surgery. Lippincott Williams and Wilkins.

Curb, JD; Aluli, Noa Emmett; Kautz JA; Petrovitch H;Knutsen SF; Knutsen R; O'Conner, Helen & O'Conner WE. 1991. Cardiovascular risk factor levels in ethnic Hawaiians. American Journal of Public Health Feb;81(2): 164-7.

Curb JD; Aluli NE; Huang BJ; Sharp DS; Rodriguez B L; Burchfield CM; & Chiu D. 1996. Hypertension in elderly Japanese Americans and adult Native Hawaiians. Public Health Report III (Suppl 2): 53-5.

Edman JL, Danko GP, Andrade N, McArdle JJ, Foster J, Glipa J. 1999. Factor structure of the CES-D (Center for Epidemiologic Studies Depression Scale) among Filipino-American adolescents. Soc Psychiatry Psychiatric Epidemiology, 34:211-215.

Goebert D & Kanoa, Kim. 1992. Injury Mortality in Hawai'i: Ethnic Diversity. The Rehab Journal 8(2). Honolulu: Rehabilitation Hospital of the Pacific and the Pacific Basin Rehabilitation Research and Training Center.

Goebert D; Birnie, Kim; Kronabel B; Percival I & Tash E. 1994. Injury Hospitalizations and Deaths in Hawai`i: Ethnic Diversity. Honolulu: Hawai`i State Department of Health.

Goebert D; Birnie, Kim; Kronabel B; Percival I & Tash E. 1994. The Geography of Injury Hospitalizations and Deaths in Hawai'i. Honolulu: Hawai'i State Department of Health.

Goebert D; Birnie, Kim; Kronabel B; Percival I & Tash E. 1994. Spanning the Ages: The magnitude of injury hospitalizations and death in Hawai'i. Honolulu: Hawai'i Department of Health, Injury Prevention & Control Program.

Goebert D; Birnie, Kim; Kronabel B; Percival I & Tash E. 1994. An overview of injury hospitalizations and death in Hawai'i. Honolulu: Hawai'i Department of Health, Injury Prevention & Control Program.

Goebert D, Birnie, Kim; Kronabel B; Percival I & Tash E. 1994. The causes and consequences of injury in Hawai'i. Honolulu: Hawai'i Department of Health, Injury Prevention & Control Program.

Goebert, D & Birnie, K. 1998. Injury and disability among Native Hawaiians. Pacific Health Dialog 5(2): 253-259.

Goebert D; Nahulu Linda; Hishinuma, E, Bell, Cathy; Yuen, Noelle; Carlton B; Andrade N; Miyamoto R & Johnson R. 2000. Cumulative effect of family environment on psychiatric symptomatology among mltiethnic adolescents. Journal of Adolescent Health 26: 34-42.

Goode RL, Burgess LPA. 1988. Bone And Cartilage Grafts in English (ed): Otolaryngology 4 (Chapter 7A): 1-14.

Goode RL, Burgess LPA. 1992. Injectable Collagen in JR Thomas, GR Holt(ed): Facial Scars: Incisions, Revision, and Camouflage: . 337-347. St. Louis: C.V. Mosby Co.

Goode RL, Burgess LPA. 1992. Collagen Implantation Technics, in JR Thomas, J Roller (ed): Cutaneous Facial Surgery: .91-95. New York: Thieme Inc.

Gotay C; Banner RO; Matsunaga DS; Hedlund N; Enos, Rachelle; Issell B & DeCambra, Ho'oipo. 2000. Impact of a culturally appropriate intervention on breast and cervical xcreening among Native Hawaiian women. Preventive Medicine 31: 529-537.

Grandinetti A; Chang H; Mau M; Curb J; Kinney EK; Sagum R; Arakaki R. 1998. Prevalence of glucose intolerance among Native Hawaiians in two rural communities. Diabetes Care 21(4):549-54.

Grandinetti A; Chang H, Chen R, Fujimoto WY, Rodriguez B & Curb JD. 1999. Prevalence of overweight and central adiposity is associated with percentage of indigenous ancestry among Native Hawaiians. International Journal of Obesity Related Metabolic Disorders 23(7): 733-7.

Grandinetti A; Kaholokula JK; Crabbe K, Kenui C; Chen R; and Chang H. 2000. Relationship between depressive symptoms and diabetes among Native Hawaiians. Psychoneuroendocrinology, Apr; 25 (3): 239-46.

Greer, Mark & Tengan, Susan. 1998. Dental caries in early childhood among Native Hawaiians. Pacific Health Dialog 5(2): 332-6.

Handy ESC; Pukui MK, Livermore K. 1934 (reprint 1985). Outline of Hawaiian Physical Therapeutics, Bishop Museum Bulletin 126. Honolulu, HI: Bishop Museum. 22(3).

Hughes CK, Tsark JA, Mokuau NK. 1996. Diet-related cancer in Native Hawaiians. Cancer Oct 1;78(7 Suppl): 1558-63.

Hughes CK, Tsark JA, Kenui C, Alexander G. 2000. Cancer research studies in Native Hawaiians and Pacific Islanders. Annals of Epidemiology10 (8): 49-60.

Judd N. 1994. Native Hawaiian traditional healing. Hawaii Medical Journal Dec;53(12):348-9.

Judd NLKM. 1997. Laau Lapaau: A Geography of Hawaiian Herbal Healing Dissertation at. University of Hawai'i at Manoa, Honolulu, Hawai'i.

Judd N. 1998. Laau Lapaau: herbal healing among contemporary Hawaiian healers. Pacific Health Dialog 5(2): 239-245.

Kaholokua JK, Grandinetti A, Crabbe KM, Chang HK, Kenui CK. 1999. Depressive symptoms and cigarette smoking among Native Hawaiians. Asian Pacific Journal of Public Health 11(2

Kinney GL. 1996. Native Hawaiian Health. Reflections 22(4): 21.

Kwee SA & Ka'anehe L. 1999. Occupational exposures and knowledge of universal precautions among medical students. Hawaii Medical Journal 58 (2).
47-149.
(4): 339-41.

Loke, Matthew & Honbo, Lynette. 2000. An update of Hawai'i's QUEST's Health Plans performance using HEDIS measures, 1997-1998. Hawai'i Medical Journal 59(11).

Look M, Sylva S, Baruffi G. 1998. The health of Hawaiian women. Pacific Health Dialog 5(2): 290-6.

Mau, Marjorie. 1998. Current status of research on diabetes mellitus and associated risk factors in Native Hawaiians. Pacific Health Dialog 5(2): 346-349.

Mau M, Grandinetti, A; Arakaki R; Chang H; Kinney, Everett; & Curb JD. 1997. The insulin resistance syndrome in Native Hawaiians. Diabetes Care 20(9): 1376-80.

Mayberry LJ; Affonso, Dyanne; Shibuya J & Clemmens D. 1999. Integrating cultural values, beliefs, and customs into pregnancy and postpartum care: lessons learned from a Hawaiian public health nursing project. Journal of Perinatal and Neonatal Nursing 13(1):15-26.

McGregor, DP & Birnie, KK. 1998. Kaho'olawe Healing. Ka'Uhane Lokahi. Honolulu: Papa Ola Lokahi.

McGregor, Davianna, Minerbi, Luciano & Matsuoka, Jon. 1998. A holistic assessment method of health and well-being for Native Hawaiian communities. Pacific Health Dialog 5(2): 361-369.

Mills, George H. 1981. Hawaiians and medicine. Hawaii Medical Journal 40(10): 272-278.

Mills, George H. 1984. Care of the elderly and chronically ill. Hawai'i Medical Journal 43(9): 302-307.

Mokuau, Noreen. 1990. The impoverishment of Native Hawaiians and the social work challenge. Health and Social Work 15(3): 235-42.

Mokuau N. 1990. A family-centered approach in native Hawaiian culture. Families in Society: The Journal of Contemporary Human Services Vol. 71 (10).

Mokuau, N (editor). 1991. Handbook of Social Services for Asian and Pacific Islanders. Connecticut: Greenwood Press.

Mokuau N; Hughes C & Tsark JA. 1995. Heart disease and associated risk factors among Hawaiians: culturally responsive strategies. Health & Social Work. 20(1): 46-51.

Prevention, Office of Minority Health & Bureau of Primary Health Care. among a native people: social work practice with Hawaiians. Social Work, 40(4):465-472.
Burgess LP & Heffner D. 1991.

National Institutes of Health. 2000. Asian American and Pacific Islander Workshops-Summary Report on Cardiovascular Health Publication No. 00-3793. Bethesda MD: National Heart, Lung, and Blood Institute, NIH, March 2000. (Contributing Authors: Aluli EA, Reyes P & Tsark J)

Native Hawaiian Health Research Project, RCMI Program. 1994. Diabetes mellitus and heart disease risk factors in Hawaiians. Hawaii Medical Journal 53(12): 340-3, 364.

Native Hawaiian Research Consortium. 1985. E Ola Mau-The Native Hawaiian Health Needs Study. Honolulu: Alu Like, Inc.:
Nishimura ST, Hishinuma ES, Miyamoto RH, Goebert DA, Johnson RC, Yuen NYC, Andrade NN. Prediction of DISC substance abuse and dependency for ethnically diverse adolescents. Journal of Substance Abuse 13 (2001) 597-607.

Odom, Sharon Ka'iulani. 1998. Hele Mai 'Ai: developing a culturally competent nutrition education program. Pacific Health Dialog 5(2): 383-5.

Office of Hawaiian Affairs. 1991. Nutrition and dental health in Hawaiians. Ka Wai Ola O OHA April 1991: 22.

Oneha MF; Magnussen L; & Feletti G. 1998. Ensuring quality nursing education in community based settings. Nurse Educator 23(1), 26-31.

O'Sullivan, Harriet Makia Awana & Lum, Kehaulani. 1999. An Investigation of the Appropriate Use of Herb-Based Products that Have Special Cultural Significance for Indigenous People: 'Awa. Honolulu HI: Papa Ola Lokahi.

Palafox Neal A & Ka'ano'i, Momi. 2000. Health Disparities among Pacific Islanders. Closing the Gap: A Newsletter of the Office of Minority Health. Bethesda MD: United States Department of Health & Human Services

Papa Ola Lokahi. 1994. Survey of AIDS Agencies and Native Hawaiian HIV/AIDS Clients. Honolulu: Papa Ola Lokahi.

Papa Ola Lokahi. 1994. First Hawaiian Health Research Conference-Conference Report and Evaluation. Honolulu: Papa Ola Lokahi.

Papa Ola Lokahi. 1996. E Ola Mau Update. Honolulu: Papa Ola Lokahi.

Johnson, David; Oyama, Neil; Le Marchand, Loic. Native Hawaiian Health Update: Mortality, Morbidity, Morbidity Outcomes and Behavioral Risks.

Greer, Mark, DMD, MPH. Native Hawaiian Oral Health.

Papa Ola Lokahi. 1998. Ka 'Uhane Lokahi, 1998 Native Hawaiian Health and Wellness Summit and Island 'Aha: Issues, Trends and General Recommendations. Honolulu: Papa Ola Lokahi.

Queen Emma Foundation. 1996. Identifying Family Violence, A community Prototype Incorporating Native Hawaiian Values and Practices. Honolulu HI: The Queen Emma Foundation.

Queen Lili'uokalani Children's Center. 1993. Hawaiian Socio-Demographic and Community Health Indicators. Honolulu HI: Queen Lili'uokalani Children's Center.

Seto D, Mokuau N, Tsark J. 1998. The interface of culture and rehabilitation for Asian and Pacific Islanders with spinal cord injuries. SCI Psychosocial Process, Jan;10(4):113-119.

Shimizu, Michele. 1990. Seasonal Abundance and Toxicity of Gambierdiscus Toxicus Adachi et Fukyo from Oahu, Hawaii. Proceedings of the Third International Conference on Ciguatera Fish Poisoning: 1990.

Shintani TT & Hughes C. 1994. Traditional diets of the Pacific and coronary heart disease. Journal of Cardiovascular Risk 1:16-20.

Shintani, Terry; Hughes C, Beckham S & O'Connor, Helen. 1991. Obesity and cardiovascular risk intervention through the ad libitum feeding of traditional Hawaiian diet. American Journal of Clinical Nutrition Jun;53(6 Suppl): 1647S-1651S.

Shintani T; Beckham S; O'Connor Helen; Hughes C; & Sato A. 1994. The Waianae Diet Program: a culturally xensitive, community-based obesity and clinical intervention program for the Native Hawaiian population. Hawaii Medical Journal May;53(5): 136-41, 147.

Shintani TT, Beckham S, Tang J, O'Conner, Helen Kanawaliwali & Hughes C. 1999. Wai'anae Diet Program: long term follow-up. Hawaii Medical Journal 58(5).

Shintani TT; Beckham S; Brown, Amy C. & O'Conner, Helen Kanawaliwali. 2001. The Hawaii Diet: ad libitum high-carbohydrate, low-fat multi-cultural diet for the reduction of chronic disease risk factors: obesity, hypertension, hypercholesterolemia, and hyperglycemia. Hawaii Medical Journal 60(3).

Silva JK; Love RK; Hobel CJ; & Magoffin DA. 1997. Maternal and umbilical cord serum immunoreactive leptin concentrations in term gestation. (Abstract) J. Soc. Gynecol. Invest. (Supplement) 4:250A.

Singh A, Noda K, & Andrade N.(1977). Fine structure of the cercariae of stellantchasmus falcatus. Journal of the Arizona Academy of Science, 12.

Smith JA; Labasky RF; Cockett, Abraham TK; Fracchia JA, Montie JE & Rowland RG. 1999. Bladder Cancer Clinical Guidelines Panel Summary Report on the management of nonmuscle invasive bladder cancer (Stages Ta, TI, AND TIS). Journal of Urology 162:1697-1701.

Spoehr H, Akau, Mahealani; Akutagawa, William; Birnie, K; Chang, Mei-Ling; Kinney, Everett; Nissanka S, Peters D, Sagum R & Soares, Dexter. 1998. Ke Ala Ola Pono: The Native Hawaiian community's effort to heal itself. Pacific Health Dialog 5(2):232-8.

Srimanunthiphol, Jun; Beddow, Ralph & Arakaki, Richard. 2000. A review of the United Kingdom Prospective Diabetes Study (UKPDS) and discussion for the implications of patient care. Hawai'i Medical Journal 59(7).

Streltzer, Jon; Rezentes, William III & Arakaki, Masa. 1996. Does acculturation influence psychosocial adaptation and well being in Native Hawaiians Int J Soc Psychiatry Spring;42(I): 28-37.

Streltzer J; Rezentes W & Arakaki M. 2000. Lack of Association of Psychosocial Variables with Natural Killer Cell Activity in a Native Hawaiian Population. Transcultural Psychiatry37(I). SI56-I59.

Tavares, Darlene N_lani. 1998. The Wai'anae Women's Health Network. Asian American and Pacific Islander Journal of Health 6(2).

Thomas WL; Cooke ES & Hammer RP. 1995. Pretreatment with a dopamine DIreceptor antagonist prevents metabolic activation by cocaine. Neuroscience Letters 196: 161-164.

Tim Sing, Patrice ML & Kamaka, Martina L. 2001. Medical school hotline. Hawai'i Medical Journal 60(7).

Titcomb, Carol L. 1990. Breast cancer and pregnancy. Hawai'i Medical Journal 49(I). Laryngoscope 107: 1066-1070.

Tsark J. 1998. Cancer in Native Hawaiians. Pacific Health Dialog 5(2): 315-327.

Tsark JU. 1998. Cancer in Native Hawaiians. Asian American and Pacific Islander Journal of Health 6(2).

Tsark JA, RK Blaisdell, E Aluli & S Finau (editors). 1998. The Health of Native Hawaiians. Pacific Health Dialog 5(2): 228-9.

Tsark J. 1993. Implications for data collection at the state and national levels. AAHF Healthy People 2000 Conference Proceedings, January 20, 1993, Honolulu, HI.

Tzikas TL, Vossoughi J, Burgess LP et al. 1996. Wound Healing: Effects of Closing Tension, Zyplast, and Platelet Derived Growth Factor. Laryngoscope 106: 322-327.

Veary, Nana. Change We Must, My Spiritual Journey. Taos, New Mexico: Medicine Bear. Visor RL, Sheridan MF, Burgess LP. 1997. Angiosarcoma of the scalp. Otolaryngol-Head and Neck Surg 117:138.Journal Sep/55(9):169-70.
Academy of Child and Adolescent Psychiatry Mar;39(3):360-7.

Yuen N, Andrade N, Nahulu L, Makini G, McDermott J, Danko G, Johnson R & Waldron J. 1996. The rate and characteristics of suicide attempters in the Native Hawaiian adolescent population. Suicide and Life-Threatening Behavior26 (1): 27.

Young, Benjamin. "A History of Imi Ho'ola." Pacific Health Dialog, Vol. 5(2); September 1998.

Uses of Hawaiian Problem-Solving Process. Institute of Culture and Communication. East-West Center. University of Hawai'i Press

Stannard, D.E. (1989). Before the Horror: The Population of Hawai'i on the eve of Western Contact. Honolulu: School of Social Science Research Institute.

Takenaka, C. (1995). A Perspective on Native Hawaiians. (Available from the Hawai'i Community Foundation, 900 Fort Street Mall, #1300, Honolulu, HI 96813)

U.S. Congress, (1988b). Native Hawaiian Health Care Act of 1988. Washington, D.C.: PL 100-579.

Wegner, E.L. (1989). The Health of Native Hawaiians, a Selective Report on Health Status and Health Care in the 1980's. Social Process in **Native Hawaiian Health References**

Aiu, P., Spoehr H. (1995). Native Hawaiian Health Initiative. Honolulu, Hawai'i: Papa Ola Lokahi. (Available from Papa Ola Lokahi 567 S. King Street, #102, Honolulu, HI 96813).

Aluli, N.E., Connor, W.E., Kahn, C., O'Connor, H.K., Petrovitch, H., Hughes, C.L. & Blaisdell, R.K. (1990). Effect of pre-Western Hawaiian diet on plasma lipids, lipoprotein and blood pressure in Native Hawaiians. Paper presented at the Hawai'i regional annual meeting of the American College of Physicians, Honolulu, HI.

Aluli, N.E. (1991). Prevalence of Obesity in a Native Hawaiian population. American Journal of Clinical Nutrition, 53, 1556S-60S.

Barringer, H., Liu, N. The Demographic, Social and Economic Status of Native Hawaiians, 1990: A Study for Alu Like, Inc. Honolulu, Hawai'i: Alu Like, Inc, 1994. Blaisdell, R.K. (1996). 1995 Update on Kanaka Maoli (Indigenous Hawaiian) Health. Asian American and Pacific Islander Journal of Health.

Braun, K.L., Look M.A., Tsark J.A.U. (1995). High Mortality rates in Native Hawaiians. Hawai'i Medical Journal; 54(9):723-729.

Bushnell, O.A. 1993). The gifts of civilization: germs and genocide in Hawai'i. Honolulu, Hawai'i; University of Hawai'i Press.

Curb, J.D. Aluli, N.E., Kautz, J.A., Petrovitch H., Knutsen S.F., Knutsen, R., O'Connor H.K., Connor, W.E. Cardiovascular risk factor levels in ethnic Hawaiians. American Journal of Public Health; 81(2):164-167.

Grossmann, B. and Shon, J. (1994). The Unfinished Health Agenda: Lessons from Hawai'i. University of Hawai'i, Honolulu, HI.

Howard, A. (1974). Ain't No Big Thing: Coping Strategies in a Hawaiian-American Community. Honolulu: The University of Hawai'i Press.

Ke Ola Mamo. (1995). Native Hawaiian Health Care System. Informational brochure. (Available from the Ke Ola Mamo, 1130 N. Nimitz Hwy, #A221, Honolulu, HI 96817)

Look, M.A. and Braun, K.L. (1995). A Mortality Study of the Hawaiian People 1910-1990. Honolulu, HI: The Queen's Health System.

Mau, M.K., Grandinettti A., Arakaki, R., Baker-Ladao, N., Chang H.K., Curb J.D. (1995). Diabetes Mellitus and Insulin Resistance Syndrome in Native Hawaiians. Diabetes; 44(SI): 174A.

McDermott, J.F., Tseng, W. and Maretzki, T.W.(1984). People and Cultures of Hawai'i: A Psychocultural Profile. John A. Burns School of Medicine and University of Hawai'i Press, Honolulu, HI.

Papa Ola Lokahi. (1992). Native Hawaiian Health Data Book. Honolulu: Papa Ola Lokahi.

Pukui, M.K., Haertig, E.W. and Lee, C.A. (1972). Nana I Ke Kumu: Look to the Source, Volumes I & II. Hui Hanai, Honolulu, HI.

Shintani, T.T., Beckham, S., O'Conner, H., Hughes, C. and Sato, A. (1994). The Wai'anae Diet Program: A Culturally Sensitive, Community-Based Obesity and Clinical Intervention Program for the Native Hawaiian Population. Hawai'i Medical Journal, 53(5), 136-147.

Shintani, T.T., Hughes, C.K., Beckham, S., O'Connor, H.K. (1991). Obesity and cardiovascular risk intervention through the ad libitum feeding of traditional Hawaiian diet. American Journal of Clinical Nutrition, 53, 1647S-51S

Shook, E.V. (1985). Ho'oponopono: Contemporary Hawai'i, 32.

APPENDIX

Terminal Progress Report "Natural Products from the Pacific" PHS Grant

GM-15198-01-03

I.   Summary:

Over 1000 species of medicinal plants, fungal cultures, marine algae, marine bacteria, and marine invertebrates have been collected, identified, studied, extracted and tested for pharmacological activity. An additional 1000 species of medicinal plants have been collected, studied, and are on hand.

A number of the pharmacologically active materials have been carried through purification procedures to a state of high specific activity, and a few to pure compounds, with partial or total structures determined.

The originally stated aims for the program were based on requested funding for seven years. The program was granted for 3 years with a six-month extension (no additional funds). These aims were:

"I.   To investigate scientifically local folklore in the Pacific Basin concerning biota useful in human medicine or thought to have other biological activity.

"2. To do the same with any Pacific biota where there are taxonomical, chemical, or even intuitive reasons for suspecting biological activity.

"3. To improve the breadth of interest and knowledge of the scientific collaborators involved.

"4. To develop useful natural product drugs for human health and welfare.

Aims 1-3 were accomplished in the collection and folklore study (of medicinal plants) of over 2000 identified species of Pacific biota and the pharmacological evaluation of over 1000 of these.

Aim 4 was not achieved, but was hardly expected to be in three years. However, we do have important and some unique biologically active materials which may well allow us to achieve aim 4 within the seven year period for which the aim was originally stated.

II.   Results:

The results will be listed in sections for each of the collaborators in the Botany, Pharmacology, and Chemistry departments.

A.   Botany, Dr. N.P. Kefford, Dept. Chairman and coordinator

I.   Dr. Melvin Lee Bristol

During a one year stay in Lefaga Bay, Western Samoa, Dr. Bristol lived with the native people, learned their language and customs, gained their confidence and respect, and consequently obtained considerable ethnobotanical information. Samples from 218 species of plants. were collected for phytochemical screening by Dr. Scheuer and pharmacological testing, and ten sets of voucher specimens in all were prepared and shipped to the Bishop Museum, Honolulu; Gray Herbarium, Cambridge, Massachusetts; U.S. National Herbarium, Washington, D.C.; Royal Botanic Garden, Kew, United Kingdom; and for his own collection.

2.   Mr. Douglas Yen (Bishop Museum)

Mr. Yen also made ethnobotanical studies, usually in co-operation with a local knowledgeable consultant. The local use of all specimens was determined, voucher specimens obtained and the identification of almost all samples was made. Over 1000 species were collected from northern Thailand, Futuna and Uvea Islands, Guam, Arno atoll in the Marshall Islands, New Britain, Gambier Islands, New Caledonia; and in the Philippines: Kakidugan, Palawan, Sulu Archipelago.

3.   Dr. Gladys Baker

Over 400 species of fungi were collected from throughout Polynesia, but primarily from the Hawaiian Islands, and purified isolates were prepared. Most have been identified and were put into the pharmacological testing program.

Several new records for. the state of Hawaii have been established. (See Publications).

I.   Dr. M. S. Doty

Over 100 species of marine algae were collected mostly from the Philippines. Depending on the availability, weights ranging from 500 g. to 20 kg. of the fresh samples were collected, cleaned, sorted, and dried. Voucher specimens were prepared and most identified.

An ecological study was made of certain algal communities at the southern tip of the island of Negros in the Philippines.

Most of the samples were extracted for testing.

An extract of *Gracilaria gigas* was found to be hypotensive by Dr. Read. Isolation work by Dr. Santos in Dr. Doty's laboratory produced a crystalline compound, m.p. 199-200°C with l max.=275 nm. Infrared spectroscopy indicated strong hydroxyl, a-ketoester or lactone, carbonyl, and hydrocarbon ($-(CH2)n$.

Chemical and pharmacological studies done on the constituents of *Caulerpa lamourouxii, C. sertularioides,* and *C. recemosa* are described in the publications listed at the end of this report with reprints enclosed.

B.   Pharmacology, Dr. T. R. Norton, coordinator

I.   Classical Pharmacology, Dr. George Read

A total of 2,084 extracts from 1,089 species were tested in rats in the "classical" Pharmacology screening program. In the accompanying table it can be seen that 521 (25%) of the extracts produced some detectable effect on the nervous, respiratory, or cardiovascular systems.

SUMMARY OF THE EFFECTS OF 2,084 EXTRACTS IN THE "CLASSICAL" PHARMACOLOGY ASSAY

Effect	Number of Extracts	Percent of 2,084
EEG Changes	1	<1
Respiratory stimulation	4	<1
ECG Changes	4	<1
Hypertension	5	<1
Hypotension	421	20
Toxic	86	4
	521	25

Only one extract was found to alter the EEG of rats. It produced "storms" of electrical activity much the same as is seen with epilepsy or pentylenetetrazol. Four extracts stimulated respiration and should be studied for their usefulness in poisoning involving respiratory depression. Another four extracts produced arrhythmias and bigeminal rhythms in the electrocardiograms of rats. Although these are signs of cardiotoxicity, these natural products should be studied because many valuable drugs used in the treatment of heart conditions show these same effects at toxic levels. Five extracts produced a rise in blood pressure which typically lasted about 5 minutes. Although this is brief, these natural products should be studied for their structures and mechanisms of action on the chance that new families of drugs and pathways might be revealed.

Hypotension was the most frequently seen effect and occurred with 421 of the extracts (20%). Because the longer acting agents would be more useful in the treatment of hypertension, it was decided to study only the 239 extracts which lowered blood pressure for more than 30 minutes. During the period of the grant, it was possible to study only a few of these; however, we can project that approximately 50% will lower blood pressure by histamine liberation, half will be effective intraperitoneally, and one-fourth will be effective orally. The following table summarizes the results of some of our preliminary studies on the characteristics of the 239 extracts which lowered blood pressure for more than 30 minutes.

SUMMARY OF PRELIMINARY STUDIES OF 239 EXTRACTS WHICH LOWERED BLOOD PRESSURE FOR MORE THAN 30 MINUTES

Action	NumberTested	Number Active	%
Histamine Liberation	38	15	39
αAdrenergic Blockade	27	0	0
Effective Intraperitoneally	119	54	45
Effective Orally	93	22	24
Heat Stable (Boiled for 5')	26	23	88

Finally, 86 of the active extracts were classified as toxic. That is, they killed the rats by disrupting all or most of the systems studied. Dilution of the extracts to reduce their response did not single out any particular system, and so these are considered to be general cytological poisons.

Below are listed the organisms which yielded the active extracts described above:

POTENTIALLY USEFUL NATURAL PRODUCTS FOUND IN THE "CLASSICAL" PHARMACOLOGY ASSAY

FRANK L. TABRAH, MD

1.   a.   1 Species yielding natural product which alters EEG

          Fungus: *Aspergillus* sp.

    b.   3 Species yielding natural products which stimulate respiration

          Fungi: *Chaetomium spirale*
                                         Polyporus sp.
          Flowering plants: *Dianthus superbus* Linn.

    c.   4 Species yielding natural products which alter ECG

          Fungi: *Aspergillus niger* van Tiegh
                                       Sclerotium rolfsii
          Flowering plants: *Morinda citrifolia*
                                       Stenolobium sp.

    d.   7 Species yielding natural products which raise blood pressure

          Fungi: *Coprinus* sp.
                                       Mucor sp.
          Flowering plants: *Pepperomia nesperomannii*
                                       Portulaca oleracea
                                     Styphelia sp.

    e.   195 Species yielding natural products which lower blood pressure for more than 30'.

        1)   Animal Kingdom (not including 3 species not yet classified)

              Coelenterates-)Cnidaria):   *Anthopleura elegantissima*
                                             Metridium senile
                                             Radianthus cookie
                                         Tealia coniacea
              Sponges-(Porifera):   *Haliclona viridis*
                                         Toxadocia violacea

        2)   Plant Kingdom (not including 27 species not yet classified)

           a)   Bacteria: *Micromonospora 23* spp. b)
           b)   Algae: *Caulerpa* sp.

           c)   Fungi:

Chaetomiaceae	*Chaetomium globosum*
Gnomoniaceae	*Glomerella cingulata*
Hypocreaceae	*Chromocrea spinulosa*
Pezizaceae	*Ascodesmis microscopia*
Pleosporiacea	*Pleospora* sp.
Sordariceae	*Podospora anserina Prussia*
Sphaeriaceae	*disperse Leptosphaerie* sp.
Xylariaceae	*Schizophyllum commune*
Agaricaceae	*Physalacria inflata Cyathus* sp.
Clavariaceae	*Fomes* sp.
Nidulariaceae	*Polyporus* sp.
Polyporacae	*Poria* sp.
	Rhodotorula mucilaginosa
Cryptococcaceae	*Alternaria* sp.
Dematiaceae	*Arthrinium* sp.
	Aureobasidium sp.
	Cladosporium herbarum
	Cladosporium sp.
	Humicola sp.
	Leptographium sp.
	Masoniella grisea
	Monosporium sp.
	Oidiodendron sp.
	Phialophora verrucosa
	Stachybotrys atra

		Zygosporium mansonii
		Zygosporium osceoides
		Calcarisporium arbusculla
		Cephalosporium sp.
	Moniliaceae	*Clonostachys* sp.
		Diheterospora sp.
		Geotrichum sp.
		Helicosporium sp.
		Monilia sp.
		Oidiodendron 2 spp.
		Paecilomyces sp.
		Penicillium citrinum
		Penicillium frequentans
		Penicillium lilacinum
		Penicillium steckii
		Penicillium 3 spp.
		Scopulariopsis brevicaulis
		Scopulariopsis 2 spp.
		Trichoderma sp.
		Verticillium sp.
		Pestalotia sp.
		Pyrenochaeta sp.
	Melanconiaceae	*Dendrographium* sp.
	Sphaeropsidaceae	*Stillbum* sp.
	Stilbellaceae	*Fusarium lateritium*
		Fusarium moniliforme
	Tuberculariaceae	*Fusarium roseum*
		Fusarium solani
		Fusarium 5 spp.
		Metarrhizium anisopliae
		Myrothecium sp.
		Weisneriomyces javanicus
		Circinella simplex
		Circinella sp.
	Mucoraceae	*Mucor niemalis*
		Mucor sphaetosporus
		Mucor 3 spp.
d)	Ferns	Asidiaceae	*Elaphoglossum* sp.
e)	Flowering Plants:	Annonaceae	*Cananga odorata*
		Apocynaceae	*Alstonia scholaris* (Linn) R. Br.
			Cerbera manghas A. Gray
			Ochrosia oppositifolia Lam.
			Tabernaemontana Subglobosa
			Trachelospermum jasminoides Lem.
		Araceae	*Amorphophallus campanulatus* (Roxburgh) Blume
			Raphidophora sp.
		Araliaceae	*Acanthopanax gracilistylus*
		Burseraceae	*Canarium decumarum* Gaertn.
		Caesalpinioideae	*Gleditsia horrida* Makio
		Campanulaceae	*Clermontia clermontioides*
		Compositae	*Cnicus spicatus* Max

Combretacea	*Terminalia* cf. *littoralis* Seeman
Connaraceae	*Agelaea borneensis*
Curcurbitaceae	*Benincasa hispida* (Thurb.) Cogn.
Cyperaceae	*Cyperus difformis*
Dipsacaceae	*Dipsacus chinensis* Bat. L.
Euphorbiaceae	*Macaranga* cf. *stipulosa*
Flacourtiaceae	*Flacourtia rukam* Zoll. and Morr.
Guttiferae	*Calophyllum inophyllum* Linn.
Iridaceae	*Moraea bicolor* Lindl.
Lardizabalaceae	*Akebia trifoliate*
Lecythidaceae	*Barringtonia asiatica* (L.) Kuntz
Leguminosae	*Acacia koa* A. Gray
	Acacia sp.
	Erythrina cf. *fusca* Louveiro
	Inocarpus edulis Forester
	Intsia bijuda (Colebr.) Kuntze
	Millettia reticulate Benth
	Phaseolus mungo Linn.
	Sophora japonica
	Strongylodon sp.
Liliaceae	*Dianella sandwicensis*
Loganiacea	*Fagraea berteriana* A. Gray
Malvaceae	*Thespesia populnea* (Linn.) Soland
Moraceae	*Ficus benjamina*
	Ficus prolixa
Myrsinaceae	*Maesa samoana*
Myrtaceae	*Eucalyptus robusta*
	Eugenia dalbergioides
Orchidaceae	*Cymbidium* "Finlay" *somanum* Lindl.
Pittosporaceae	*Pittosporum* sp.
Plantaginaceae	*Plantago major* Linn.
Portulacaceae	*Portulaca grandiflora* Hook
Proteaceae	*Macadamia integrifolia*
Ranunculaceae	*Paeonia albiflora*
Rhamnaceae	*Colubrina asiatica* (L.) Brongn.
Rosaceae	*Chaenomeles sinensis* (Thouin) Koehne
Rubiaceae	*Hedyotis kingiana*
	Morinda citrifolia
Rutaceae	*Evodia ternata*
Santalaceae	*Santalum freycinetianum* Gaudich.
Simaroubaceae	*Simarouba glauca* DC.
Solaneaceae	*Solanum macranthum* Hook
Sterculiaceae	*Kleinhovia hospita* Linn.
Umbelliferae	*Siler divaricatum* Benth. and Hook.
Verbenaceae	*Premna conjesta*
	Premna taitensis Schauer
Vitaceae	*Leea* sp.

2,   <u>Columbia S. K. Virus Screening</u>, Mrs. M. Kashiwagi

This test was done in mice as described by W. C. Cuting, *et al.* (Proc. Soc. Exp. Biol., N.Y. <u>120</u>, 330-333 (1965)). During the first two years of the program, 767 extracts of natural products were screened. Only one, *Vibrio parhaemolyticus*, a marine bacterium collected in the Pacific Ocean near Hawaii by Dr. Kaare Gunderson has shown repeatable activity. The data showing activity is substantial for the crude extracts. However, many attempts at purification using gentle techniques (Sephadex), dialysis, even lyophilization, have caused partial or complete loss of activity. Because of the poor batting average, this test was dropped near the end of 1969 in favor of more testing capacity for Ehrlich ascites tumor.

3.   <u>Ehrlich Ascites Screening & Evaluation, Mrs. M. Kashiwagi and Dr. T. R. Norton</u>

A total of 1379 extracts of 868 different species of biota were screened for activity against Ehrlich ascites tumor in mice. The breakdown according to types was:

		Species	Extracts
a.	Plants		
	Terrestrial	265	461
	Marine algal	93	144
b.	Animals		
	Marine	54	59
c.	Bacteria		
	Marine (cultures)	45	45
d.	Fungi		
	Wild	6	6
	Cultured	398	657
e.	Pure chemical	7	7
	TOTAL	868	1379

Extracts of the following species showed a minimum of doubling the mean survival time of mice injected i.p. with Ehrlich ascites tumor cells:

a. Terrestrial plants:

Ficus tinctoria Forst.
Iroro philipinensis
Melochia sp.

b. Fungi (cultured):

Cylindrocarpon lucidum
Calonectria sp.

c. Marine invertebrates:

Stoichactis kenti (?) Hand (anemone)
Cephaea conifera (jellyfish)
Nephthya sp. (soft coral)
Lanice conchilega (annelid)
Reteterebella queenslandia (annelid)
Aurelia labiata (jellyfish)
Anthopleura elegantissima (anemone)
Anthopleura xanthogrammica (anemone)
Palythoa psamnophilia (zoanthid)
Zoanthu pacificus (zoanthid)
Radianthus cookie (anemone)

The first five of the marine invertebrates were first collected and extracted by Dr. F. L. Tabrah, clinical professor of Pharmacology (UH), and arrangements were made by him for the collection of the *Anthopleura* species by Mrs. Daphne Dunn of the Bodega Bay Marine Station, California.

It is interesting to note that extracts of none of the marine algae and marine bacteria showed activity; 1% of the plants and 0.5% of the cultured fungi showed activity; while an impressive 20% of the marine animals showed high activity against Ehrlich ascites tumor.

Evaluation studies have shown that a purified fraction from *S. kenti* cures Ehrlich ascites (survival >6 mos.), acts systemically (drug i.p., EA cells sub-cu. and vice versa), is effective when drug is given 36 hrs. prior to EA inoculation, is effective when drug is given 4 days after EA inoculation, and is effective with only two drug doses (in screening 20 doses over 10 days given).

4. Antimicrobial Testing, Dr. O. Bushnell

Screening against II mycobacteria and seven Gram positive and Gram negative bacteria was carried out *in vitro* with II60 extracts of 660 species of biota. Some 30 extracts showed repeatable inhibition of at least two strains of bacteria.

5. Central Nervous System Effects, S. Shibata

Some 100 extracts were selected because they had exhibited some effects in either the cancer screening in mice or in the classical pharmacology in rats. Effects looked for in mice were spontaneous motor activity, anticonvulsant activity, fighting behavior, sedative activity, relation to dimethamphetamine effect, hypothermic activity and analgesic activity, effects upon conditioned responses, effect on blood pressure, acute toxicity, and paralyzing activity.

Several convulsants, several muscle relaxants, many inhibitors of spontaneous motor ac6tivity, several hypothermics and many sedatives were found.

Detailed evaluation was carried out on extracts of:

Acanthaster planci (starfish)—hypothermia, vascular smooth muscle relaxation, hypotension (G. Read) and a 24% increase ($p<0.05$) in barbiturate sleep time. The purified fraction was found to be a histamine liberator.

Stoichactis kenti(?) (anemone). A pure fraction from this has been studied in depth (Ph.D. thesis for Prasad Turlapaty). Briefly, it was found that a central adrenergic mechanism plays the major role in the stimulant activity (fighting behavior and convulsions) and requires the presence of tissue catecholamine and catecholamine synthesis. Interactions with cholinergic and anticholinergic drugs support this hypothesis. It is somewhat like amphetamine in mechanism of action.

Anthopleura xanthogrammica (anemone). A purified fraction of this extract showed a strong positive inotropic effect, reversed arrhythmias, and stimulated normal heart action after ouabain induced cardiac arrest in isolated rabbit heart.

Anthopleura elegantissima (anemone). Extracts of this animal appear to contain the same active component as *A. xanthogrammica.*

6. <u>Antifertility, Dr. A. deS. Matsui and Dr. W. C. Cutting</u>

Two hundred extracts of natural products were screened using the method described in W. C. Cutting, *et al.*, Med. .Pharm. exp. <u>15</u>, 7-16 (1966). Of these, 29 showed a decrease in fertility in two or more subsequent runs. About half were toxic at the effective dose (wt. loss and appearance) and effectiveness was probably related to toxicity. None of the effective agents suppressed the estrus cycle, suggesting non-inhibition of pituitary gonadotropin. Most produced their effect between ovulation and implantation. One of the most effective extracts comes from *Dianthus superbus* (which is also hypotensive).

This screening program was terminated at the end of 1968, when Dr. Matsui left the University of Hawaii. Dr. Cutting spent some time in 1969 in attempts to isolate the active constituent, but it appears quite sensitive to decomposition as all fractions obtained had less activity than the crude extract. The project was dropped.

7.   Propagation of Fungus Cultures,. Dr. J. F. Lenney

Some 425 fungal isolates obtained from Dr. Baker's group were successfully propagated and extractions made of both the mycelia and the broth (850 extracts). Anti-cancer, hypotensive, and antibacterial activity of a number of these has been found.

8.   Rauscher Virus, MCDV-12 Ascites Tumor, and Walker Tumor, Dr. P. E. Yoder

About 20 extracts were tested against Rauscher, 100 in the ascites and 4 in Walker. The only activity of significance was that of the extract of *Lanice conchilega* on Rauscher. This extract also showed activity against Ehrlich ascites tumor (see B-3). This part of the program was terminated at the end of 1968.

9.   Purification of Biologically Active Extracts Dr. T. R. Norton, Dr. Prasad Turlapaty (Ph.D., 12/71), Mrs. M. Kashiwagi

HEALTHCARE HAWAII STYLE

a. Extracts found active against Ehrlich ascites tumor.

1) *Lanice conchilega* (marine annelid from Hawaii).

The crude extract shows excellent activity in Ehrlich ascites tumor, significant activity in Rauscher and marginal activity in P-388 (NCI). The crude extract was dialyzed, the retentate treated with pronase and redialyzed. The retentate was active at 1 mg./dose (per 28 g. mouse) compared to 17 mg./dose of crude extract. A sample of this pronase treated fraction has been submitted to NCI for further testing in P-388. Further isolation work was abandoned because of the difficulty in collection of adequate quantities of specimens and the relatively low specific activity compared to the related annelid, *Reteterebella queers landia* below.

2) *Reteterebella queenslandia* (marine annelid from Australia)

One kilogram wet weight of tentacles has been processed as follows:

The tentacles were homogenized with 30% EtOH, centrifuged, evaporated, and dialyzed. The lyophilized retentate was defatted with $CHCl_3$ and subjected to gel permeation chromatography on Sephadex G-75 twice. The fraction at Ve/Vo=1.4-1.85 had an activity max. at Ve/Vo=1.76. A total of 600 mg. is on hand active at 7 µg./dose (per 28 g. mouse). About 50% of the crude extract activity was obtained while eliminating 99.4% of the original wet weight of impurities. This fraction is not deactivated by pronase treatment. The molecular weight is ca. 8000 based on Ve/Vo values on G-50 and G-75.

3) *Nepthya* sp. (soft coral from Australia)

Preliminary separation work using a procedure similar to above with 900 g. wet wt. of coral, except that G-50 was used. The fraction at Ve/Vo 0.79-1.74 was active at 0.15 mg./dose. About 98% of the activity was recovered while eliminating 98.5% of the original wet weight of impurities.

4) *Stoichactis kenti(?)** (sea anemone from Tahiti)

A 14-step purification procedure was worked out prior to the termination of this grant. Since the termination some 8 kg. wet weight of anemones has been processed to a defatted dialysis retentate (62 g.) active at 100 µg./dose.

About 1/8 of this retentate has been chromatographed and deionized with MB-1 resin to give some 725 mg. of lyophilized material active at 12 µg./dose. This procedure recovers about 68% of the activity while removing 99.93% of the original wet weight of impurities. Enough material is on hand for 400,000 mouse doses.

Also since the termination of this grant further chromatography has given a crystalline product active at 1 µg./dose.

* Identified by Dr. Cadet Hand at Bodega Bay Marine Station as "certainly *Stoichactis* and most probably *S. kenti.*"

b. <u>A CNS Stimulant.</u> *Stoichactis kenti(?)*

From the same animal as in a-4) a toxic fraction (the pharmacology of which is described in B-5) was isolated and since the termination of this grant over 0.5 g. of the pure substance has been isolated. It is a basic polypeptide containing 17 different amino-acids all identified using an amino acid analyzer and all are neutral or basic.

c. <u>A Heart Stimulant.</u> *Anthopleura xanthogrammica*

The pharmacology of this anemone extract is mentioned in section B-5. A purified fraction was obtained by dialysis and G-50 fractionation of the defatted retentate. The active fraction is eluted at Ve/Vo of about 2.5 (U.V. abs. peak, 280 nm). If an approximate molecular weight of 1000 is assumed (probably higher), this fraction reverses 10^{-4} molar ouabain cardiac arrest at *10* molar concentration. It also exhibits the positive inotropic effect at the same concentration.

d. <u>Antihypertensives</u>

1) *Acacia koa* Gray (Leguminosae, indigenous to Hawaii)

The hot water extract of the leaves is hypotensive (>2 hrs.) i.v. in anesthetized rats, at 166 mg./kg. The lyophilized extract was dissolved in McOH, filtered and active solids precipitated by diluting the MeOH 1/1. with 2-propanol. Caffeine added to an aqueous solution of this solid removed the tannins, and the filtrate was deionized with MB-1 resin and dialyzed. The active retentate was resolved by gel chromatography on G-25 into two fractions with 280 nm U.V. abs. max at Ve/Vo=1.55 and 1.78. These individual fractions had 25% of the specific activity that the recombination of them exhibited indicating synergism. The combination was active at 1.6 mg./kg. An aqueous solution gives stable foam and causes rapid red cell lysis indicating a saponin. These fractions were given to Dr. Scheuer for further purification and characterization.

2) *Ficus benjamina L.* (Moraceae, introduced into Hawaii from India)

The lyophilized crude 60% EtOH extract was treated with MeOH and the filtrate was diluted with CCl_4 to give an 8/3 ratio of CCl /MeOH. The active material precipitated. It was then deionized with MB-1 and chromatographed on G-15. A broad band at Ve/Vo 1.5-3.2 gives a solid active at 50 mg./kg. It shows negative alkaloid and positive phenolic tests. This was given to Dr. Scheuer for further purification and characterization.

3) *Moraea bicolor* Lindl. (Iridacea, introduced into Hawaii from Africa)

A 60% EtOH extract of the rhizomes was active at 140 mg./kg. Dialysis gives a retentate active at 17 mg./kg. The active substance is precipitated from water by caffeine and will not move on Sephadex indicating possibly a polyphenolic or tannin-like substance.

4) *Simarouba glauca* (Simaroubaceae, introduced into Hawaii from Tropical America)

After extraction of the leaves with methylene chloride, the marc was dried and extracted with 60% EdOH. After EtOH removal, the aqueous solution was dialyzed and the diffusate treated with nylon powder hot (MgO removes activity) and the filtrate separated on G-25. The fraction at Ve/Vo=1.45-1.70 was evaporated to 100 mg./ml. concentration and the addition of 2-propanol precipitated solids active at *ca.* 15 mg./kg. This material was given to Dr. Sheuer for further purification work.

5) *Solanum macrathum* Dun. (Solanaceae, introduced into Hwaii from Brazil)

Yellow crystalline needle clusters were obtained and found to be hypotensive at <1 mg./kg. The dried leaves were extracted (Soxhlet) with $CHCl_3$ and the dried marc extracted with MeOH. The MeOH extract was evaporated with H_2O until the MeOH was gone. The ppt. which formed (pH 4.6) was separated and it dissolved readily in 1M NH_3. The solution was evaporated and at pH 9 the aqueous solution was extracted with n-BuOH. The n-BuOH was evaporated to remove the water. On cooling a solid deposited. It was dialyzed and the retentate separated on Sephadex G-25. The active fraction was chromatographed on Cellex-D (anion exchange pH 7.0, 0.01M PO_4) and a pure fraction once more passed through G-25 to remove phosphate and give a fraction with a clean peak (U.V. 280 nm) at Ve/Vo=2.8. On evaporation of this fraction clean yellow clusters of needles deposited. These were strongly hypotensive at <1.0 mg./kg.

6) *Acanthaster planci* (Crown of Thorns starfish – Molokai)

Both the spines and the body gave active extracts. A 95% EtOH extract was evaporated with water to give an aqueous solution (centrifuged ppt. discarded). The aqueous solution was sequentially extracted with diethyl ether and benzene, and the organic layers discarded. Then at pH 4.5 and in 5% NaCl the active portion was extracted by n-BuOH. The addition of acetone precipitated an active solid which was dissolved in water and dialyzed. The retentate was lyophilized to give a solid active at 15 mg/kg. TLC with n-BuOH/HOAc/H_2O in 12/3/5 proportions gave three distinct spots at R_f=0.64, 0.72, and 0.78, all showing positive saponin spot tests with phosphotungstic acid. A solution of the solid caused rapid hemolysis of red cells. The material was found to be a histamine liberator and further pharmacological work was terminated.

C. Chemistry, Dr. Paul J. Scheuer, coordinator, Dr. R. E. Moore

1. Dr. Scheuer's Research

   a. Summary Statement

   Our section of the program was charged

   1) with the preparation of primary extracts from sample collections in Hawaii and elsewhere in the Pacific or terrestrial and marine plants to render them suitable for pharmacolocigal screening; and

   2) with structural elucidation of some of the materials that were found active in the screening program.

   We carried out the grinding and extracting as far as available manpower resources permitted. However, several hundred samples have remained unprocessed at the termination of the program.

   We performed separation and isolation work for four materials that were found active in the screening program.

   We investigated two endemic species of the plant family Lobeliaceae, which are related to a rare species that had shown activity in the screening program.

We carried out isolation and purification work on the toxin of a marine gastropod mollusk.

b. Results

1) Preliminary separations were performed on Preliminary separations were performed on Preliminary separations were performed on

  a) the marine annelid *Lanice conchilega*

  b) the endemic tree *Acacia koa*

  c) the introduced ornamental *Ficus benjamina*

2. Isolation and characterization was carried out on the extract from the introduced tree *Barringtonia asiatica*. The active fraction contains triterpenoids related to, or identical with, the known barrigenols.

3. The endemic lobeliaceous shrub *Clermontia kakeana* was found to contain

  a) the alkaloid 8-ethylnorlobelone

  b) the triterpenoid ursolic acid

4. One gram of racemic 8-ethylnorlobelone hydrochloride was synthesized for the pharmacology program.

5. From the endemic shrub *Lobelia yuccoides* we had previously isolated an alkaloid. We synthesized its principal degradation product and made a number of unsuccessful attempts to synthesize the alkaloid itself.

b. List of Results:

Isolation and structure determination of two highly unsaturated hydrocarbons from Hawaiian *Dictyopteris*.

Isolation and structure determinations of four novel sulfur compounds from Hawaiian *Dictyopteris*.

Synthesis of model compounds related to a degradation product of palytoxin, a highly toxic substance from a coelenterate.

The secondary spines of sea urchins of the genus *Echinothrix* do not possess a toxin as previously reported.

Tri-2-n-butoxyethyl phosphate, a plasticizer used chiefly in synthetic rubber, has been found in seaweed (*Dictyopteris*) and marine animals (*Palythoa*).

III. Publications and Planned Publications

There are 20 publications and papers in press, 4 submitted, 3 in preparation, and 30 planned that have resulted from this grant.

I. Dr. Gladys Baker

(1) Kohlmeyer, Jan, Marine Fungi of Hawaii including the New Genus *Heliascus, Can. J. Bot.* 47 (9), 1469-1487 (1969).

(2) Kohlmeyer, Jan, Mangrove Fungi, *Trans. Brit. Mycol. Soc.,* 53 (2), 237-250 (1969).

(3) Goos, R. D., Phalloid Fungi in Hawaii, *Pacifica Sci.* XXIV (2), 282-287 (1970).

(4) Goos, R. D., *In vitro* Sporlation in *Actinospora megalospora, Trans. Br. Mycol. Soc.* 55 (2), 335-337 (1970).

(5) Goos, R. D., A New Genus of the *Hythomycetes* from Hawaii, *Mycologia* 62 (1), 171-175 (1970).

(6) Goos, R. D., *Listeromyces* species *insignis* Refound, *Mycologia* 63 (2), 213-218 (1971).

(7) Dring, D. M., J. Meeker and R. Goos, *Claythrus oahuensis*, a New Species from Hawaii, *Mycologia* 63 (4), 893-897 (1971).

2. <u>Dr. M. S. Doty</u>

(8) Santos, G. A. and M. S. Doty, Caulerpa as Food in the Philippines, *Philippine Agriculturist* <u>52</u>, 477-482 (1969).

(9) Doty, M. S. and G. A. Santos, Transfer of Toxic Algal Substances in Marine Food Chains, *Pacific Sci.* <u>24</u>, 351-355 (1970).

(10) Santos, G. A., Caulerpin, a New Red Pigment from Green Algae of the Genus *Caulerpa*, *J. Chem. Soc.* <u>1970</u>, 842-843.

(11) Santos, G. A. and M. S. Doty, Constituents of the Green Alga *Caulerpa lamourouxii*, *Lloydia* <u>34</u>, 88-90 (1971).

3. Special Project by M. Weiner in Botany

(12) Weiner, M. A., Notes on Some Medicinal Plants of Fiji, *Econ. Bot.* <u>24</u>, 279-282 (1970).

4. <u>Dr George W. Read</u>

(13) Read, G. W., G. S. Naguwa, J. J. Wigington, and J. F. Lenney, A Histamine Liberator in the Tannin Fraction of the Eucalypts, *Lloydia* <u>33</u>, 461-471 (1970).

(14) Read, G. W. and J. F. Lenney, Molecular Weight Studies n the Active Constituents of Compound 48/80, *J. Med. Chem.*, in press.

5. Dr. A. deS. Matsui and Dr. W. C. Cutting

(15) Matsui, deS., A. S. Hoskin, M. Kashiwagi, B. W. Agu-da, B. E. Zegart, T. R. Norton and W. C. Cutting, A Survey of Natural Products from Hawaii and Other Areas of the Pacific for an Antifertility Effect in Mice, *Int. J. Clin. Pharmacol., Ther. & Tox.* 5 (1), 65-69 (1971).

(16) Matsui, deS., A. J. Rogers, Y. K. Woo, S. Hoskin, M. Kashiwagi, T. R. Norton and W. C. Cutting, Antifertility Effect of Crude Extracts of *Dianthus superbus* in Mice, *Int. J. Clin. Pharmacol., Ther. & Tox.*4 (2), 366-370 (1969)

(17) Tabrah, F. L., M. Kashiwagi, and T. R. Norton, Inhibition of Tumor Growth by *Lanice conchilega* Tentacle Extracts, *Science* 170, 181-3 (1970).

(18) Tabrah, F. L., M. Kashiwagi, and T. R. Norton, Antitumor Effect in Mice of Four Coelenterate Extracts, *Int. J. Clin. Pharmacol., Ther. & Tox.* 6 (1), in press.

6. Dr. R. E. Moore

(19) Pettus, J. A., Jr. and R. E. Moore, Isolation and Structure Determination of an Undeca-1, 3, 5, 8-tetraene and Dictyopterene B from Algae of the Genus *Dictyopteris, Chem. Commun.* 1970, 1093.

(20) Roller, P., K. Au and R. E. Moore, Isolation of S-(3-Oxoundecyl) Thioacetate, Bis-(3-oxoundecyl) Disulfide, (-)-3-Hexyl-4, 5-dithiacycloheptanone, and S-(trans-3-Oxoundec-4-enyl) Thioacetate from *Dictyopteris, Chem. Commun.* 1971, 503.

INDEX

"fig" identifies pictures.

HHSC. *See* Hawaii Health Systems Corporation (HHSC)
HIFA. *See* Health Insurance Flexibility and Accountability
    Initiative (HIFA)
Hill-Burton legislation, 84
Hillebrand, Dr. William, 17–18, 20, 29, 31 fig, 45
Hilo, 37, 55
    Clinic, 128
    Drug Building, 60 fig
    Group Practice, 128
    Hospital, 77, 79, 95, 116, 130
    Kutsanai, Dr. Toshio, 82
    massacre (1938), 65
    Matsumura Japanese Hospital, 80–81 fig
Hilo Drug Building, 60 fig
Hilo hospital, 77, 79, 130
HMSA. *See* Hawaii Medical Service Association (HMSA)
Hoffman, Dr. Edward, 13
Honolulu
    Bishop Museum, 90
    Board of Health Building, 17 fig
    depopulation of, 14
    Hospital, 66, 126
    Kapiolani Park, 13, 16 fig
    Koloa, 5, 77
    Queen's Hospital, 23 fig, 50
    rate increase, hospital, 22 fig
    smallpox epidemic (1853), 13–21
Honolulu Advertiser, 41–42
Honomu plantation, 47
Hooper, Dr. William, 5–6
hospital
    acute care, 128, 132

Index by Clive Pyne
www.cpynebookindexing.com/

Made in the USA